Learning Dynamic Spatial Relations

Andreas Bihlmaier

Learning Dynamic Spatial Relations

The Case of a Knowledge-based Endoscopic Camera Guidance Robot

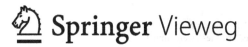 Springer Vieweg

Andreas Bihlmaier
Karlsruhe, Germany

PhD Thesis, Karlsruhe Institute of Technology (KIT), 2016

ISBN 978-3-658-14913-0   ISBN 978-3-658-14914-7 (eBook)
DOI 10.1007/978-3-658-14914-7

Library of Congress Control Number: 2016946311

Springer Vieweg

Printed on acid-free paper

This Springer Vieweg imprint is published by Springer Nature
The registered company is Springer Fachmedien Wiesbaden GmbH

For puiu

Acknowledgement

A number of people beyond the author of this PhD thesis have been essential to achieve the results presented here. My first "Thank You" is directed to Prof. Heinz Wörn and Prof. Beat Müller not only for their guidance and advice, but without them there would not even have been a research project to start my work on. In this context, I also want to acknowledge everyone involved in writing the Sonderforschungsbereich/Transregio 125 "Cognition-Guided Surgery"[1] project proposal, in particular Oliver Weede, who set the goal within the project to research into autonomous endoscope guidance.

Thanks to everybody involved into the SFB/Transregio 125 project. A special acknowledgement is mandatory for Hannes Kenngott, Martin Wagner and Patrick Mietkowski: Without your help nothing would have been possible. No interdisciplinary papers on surgical robotics would have been written; no prizes would have been won.

The other important context was the Institute for Anthropomatics and Robotics – Intelligent Process Control and Robotics (IAR-IPR), which has a great culture of informal interactions, sincere criticism and mutual support, thanks to everybody there. Not least to the secretaries, without whom there would be no time left to do research. Furthermore, a big thanks to all undergraduates for their contributions.

Finally, I am grateful to my wife, my family and all dear friends for their support and enduring a PhD student's work-life balance that often has too much weight in the work pan.

Karlsruhe   Andreas Bihlmaier

[1]Funded by the Deutsche Forschungsgemeinschaft (DFG) and undertaken as a cooperation by the University Hospital Heidelberg, the Karlsruhe Institute of Technology (KIT) and the German Cancer Research Center (DKFZ).

Contents

Glossary

API Application Programming Interface.

CQC Camera Quality Classifier.

CT Computed Tomography.

Degree of freedom is used to describe the number of independent motions of a system. An unconnected rigid body has six degrees of freedom (DoF), three translations and three rotations. In a serial kinematic chain, the number of joints corresponds to the number of DoF. These can be less than the six required DoF to freely position a body in space (kinematic deficiency) or more (kinematic redundancy)
.

DoF Degree of freedom.

FLS Fundamentals of Laparoscopic Surgery.

FRI Fast Research Interface.

Fundamentals of Laparoscopic Surgery is an educational program comprising the fundamental knowledge and technical skills for laparoscopic surgery. The manual tasks are often utilized for various benchmarks. .

GUI Graphical User Interface.

HMI Human-Machine Interface.

HMM Hiden Markov Models.

HRI Human-Robot Interaction.

IDL Interface Description Language.

LWR Light Weight Robot.

MIS Minimally-Invasive Surgery.

ML Machine Learning.

MRI Magnetic Resonance Imaging.

OR Operating Room.

PTP Point-To-Point.

RCM Remote Center-of-Motion.

Real-Time is used in different contexts in computer science. Often it merely refers the capability to process (streaming) data "fast enough", e.g. at sensor rate or for interactive use. This is the case for "real-time rendering". However, in the context of robotics, real-time usually refers to real-time computing/systems. In this context, a real-time system must not only guarantee the logical correctness of its results, but also that responses happen at a specified time (temporal correctness). .

RGB Red Green Blue.

RGB-D Red Green Blue & Depth.

ROS Robot Operating System.

RPC Remote Procedure Call.

RT Real-Time.

SDF Simulation Description Format.

TLX Task Load Index.

URDF Unified Robot Description Format.

XML Extensibe Markup Language.

1 Introduction

The aim of this thesis is to describe novel methods that facilitate autonomous robotic endoscope assistance, which is derived from actual surgical know-how. In minimally-invasive surgery (MIS), the surgeon has to rely on an assistant to guide the endoscope camera for him in order to get a view at the surgical site. Given the many issues that arise from this situation, motorized endoscope holders appeared early in the short history of MIS. Nevertheless, even today's assistance systems are still based on the paradigm of manual control by the surgeon. Even research systems looking to increase the autonomy of the endoscope robots have largely focused on simple control rules such as directly following the instruments. The system detailed in this thesis combines modelling of spatial relations with machine learning techniques in order to directly acquire the complex and situation-dependent relation between endoscope position and surgical action. A generic model of endoscope motions is predefined. However, the specific endoscope positions best suited to the surgical task are learned from concrete actions of a camera assistant utilizing his surgical know-how.

Due to the interdisciplinary nature of this task, situated between computer science and surgery, contributions from both sciences are essential. Although it is impossible to clearly separate one field from the other in this task, the work at hand provides the technical perspective of the system from a robotics and computer science point of view.

The major contributions to the field of medical robotics, which represent the core of this thesis are:

- The first knowledge-based endoscopic camera guidance system with a performance on the level of a human assistant (interdisciplinary contribution).

- A unified model and algorithm pipeline for representing, learning and moving a robot according to dynamic spatial relationships (disciplinary contribution).

Since it is important to understand the overall scenario in which endoscopic camera guidance plays an important role, some brief background information on minimally-invasive surgery will be provided in the following section. This will be followed by a short primer on surgical robotics and knowledge-based cognitive systems. At the end of this chapter an overview of the overall thesis is provided.

1.1 Minimally-Invasive Surgery

1.1.1 A new kind of surgery

Minimally-invasive Surgery (MIS) in the abdomen[1] refers to surgical procedures which are performed through very small incisions with long tubular instruments (Fig. 1.1). A trocar is inserted into each incision and fixed in place with a few stitches. The trocar allows to insert an instrument through it while at the same time creating a tight seal with the abdominal wall. The patient's abdomen is then inflated with carbon dioxide (CO2) gas to create an artificial pneumoperitoneum that separates the abdominal wall from the organs inside (Fig. 1.2). In order to get a view from the inside of the patient's abdominal cavity, an endoscope is inserted through one of the trocars. The endoscope (Fig. 1.3a) consists of rod lenses as optics that transport an image to a camera located outside of the patient. Fiber optics on the perimeter of the endoscope transmit light, which illuminates the abdominal cavity. The most common MIS instruments (Fig. 1.3b) are grasper, scissors, electrocautery and stapler.

MIS in its modern form has only been around since 1985 when the first laparoscopic cholecystectomy[2] was performed [1]. Yet, the laparoscopic procedure quickly gained acceptance in the surgical

---

[1]Visceral surgery.
[2]Removal of the gallbladder by surgery.

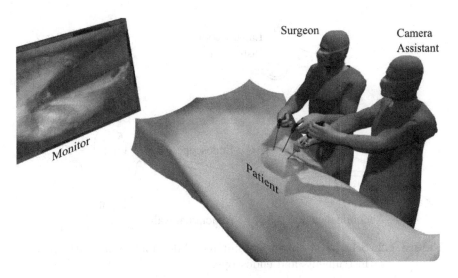

Figure 1.1: Outline of operating room, medical staff, patient and monitor in minimally-invasive surgery.

community [2]. This was mainly driven by early results [3] showing less complications and a reduced mortality rate, although an increase in the rate of common bile duct injury. Also soft factors play an important role, such as a shortened hospital stay and better cosmetic results due to less scarring. From a technical point of view, the availability of sufficiently small and cheap video cameras with good enough light sensitivity and resolution paved the way for MIS. Only through advanced technologies was it possible to bring the laparoscopic view onto a screen, which allowed tolerable working conditions. More information on the early history of laparoscopic surgery can be found in the overview by Lau et al. [4].

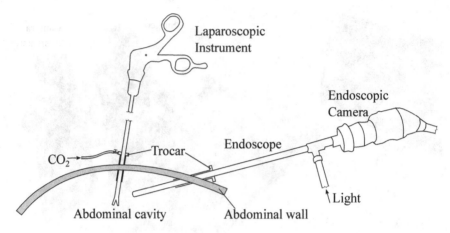

Figure 1.2: Schematic drawing of inflated abdominal cavity with trocars, instruments and endoscope.

1.1.2 Ergonomic Challenges

However, the new method also had some significant drawbacks, especially for the surgeon. Compared to open surgery, the hand-eye coordination becomes much more difficult [5][6]. Therefore, MIS as a surgical technique requires additional motor skills training [7]. Instead of directly looking at his own hands, the surgeon has to look away from the operating site towards the endoscope monitor (Fig. 1.1).

This additional level of indirection compared to open surgery can be expressed through interaction models. Figure 1.4 illustrates the differences in a block diagram following Stassen et al. [8]. Furthermore, the so called fulcrum effect, i.e. the mirroring of motion together with motion scaling depending on instrument insertion depth, is known to increase the difficulty in MIS [9]. Zheng et al. [10] evaluated the mental workload of 12 novice and 9 expert surgeons during complex tasks such as laparoscopic suturing. The Fundamentals of Laparoscopic Surgery (FLS) scoring system [11] was used to asses the sutures. In parallel to performing the suturing task, the participants had to attend to a visual detection task. Error rates of this task were used as further

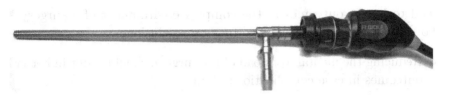

(a) Image of an endoscope with camera and light source attached.

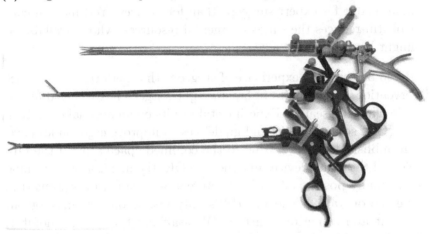

(b) A grasper, scissors and stapler for MIS with rigid bodies and markers for optical tracking.

Figure 1.3: Minimally-invasive instruments for laparoscopy.

scores. As expected, metrics for the suture tasked strongly correlated with the laparoscopic experience of the surgeon. The expert surgeons were also able to better attend to the visual detection in parallel. As pointed out by the authors, mental resources are a finite resource, through practice more resources are freed, e.g. through motor skill automaticity, and can be allocated to secondary tasks: "This explains why experienced surgeons are able to notice abnormal events in the operating room (OR), respond to events faster, and initiate preemptive maneuvers better than novice surgeons. The spare mental resource provides the foundation for situation awareness and perhaps would

lead to better outcomes in the complex environment of a surgery."
For the topic of this thesis, two further conclusions can be drawn:

- Reducing the mental workload of the surgeon should result in better
  outcomes in case complications occur.

- Manual control of a motorized endoscope holder by the surgeon is
  more viable for expert surgeons than for novices. Yet, manual control still reduces the surgeon's mental resources, whose availability
  might benefit the patient.

Based on the daily experience of surgeons that perform a lot of MIS
interventions, ergonomics in laparoscopic surgery has received attention in clinical research. Experimental results on an optimal operating
room (OR) setup for MIS and guidelines to improve ergonomics have
been published [12]. Yet, due to the confined space around the OR
table and the many devices in a modern OR, the monitor often cannot
be optimally positioned for both surgeon and camera assistant [13].
Since the operating field in MIS is only visible on-screen, surgeon,
assistant and sometimes further OR staff must view the monitor.
Thus, in combination with the required arm positions, the OR staff
has to take unfavorable postures (Fig. 1.5).

These postures have to be maintained for an extended period of
time over the course of the intervention [14]. This is problematic
because the constant head rotation, for example, can induce fatigue
and cause neck pain or headaches. Surveys state [15] that as much
as 84% of surgeons consider the working posture uncomfortable or
even painful. This ergonomic risk [16] does not only apply to the
surgeon, but also to the camera assistant. It is quite common that
either the camera assistant or the surgeon could stand in an adequate
posture individually, but not both at the same time because of spatial
constraints at the OR table. Moran [17] even states that "the most
frustrating aspect of these types of [laparoscopic] surgeries comes from
difficulties in interacting with the camera operator."

Beyond the negative effects on the OR staff, a good view on the
operating field has an impact on the surgical outcome. Studies by

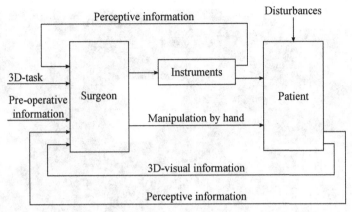

(a) Open surgery: Direct manipulation and direct visual observation.

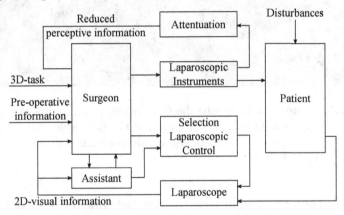

(b) Minimally-invasive surgery: Indirect manipulation via instruments and indirect visual observation via laparoscope.

Figure 1.4: Block diagrams of surgeon-patient interaction (Stassen et al. [8]).

Hanna et al. [18] [19] provide clear evidence that the endoscopic view has a direct impact on the laparoscopic task performance. This pertains to both location of the monitor showing the endoscopic image and the intracorporeal spatial relation between endoscope and instruments. The ideal monitor position was found to be as close as

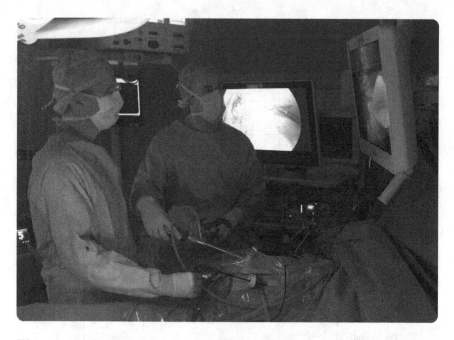

Figure 1.5: Exemplary view into the OR during a minimally-invasive
surgery. The tight space around the OR table often requires
the staff to take on unergonomic postures over an extended
period of time.

possible in the line of sight towards the instruments [19]. However,
the second influence on the surgical performance, position of the
endoscope relative to operating area and instruments, is much more
relevant to this thesis. Target-to-endoscope distance and manipulation
angle of instruments are shown to have a significant influence on the
task performance of endoscopic knot tying [18]. The direction of
view was not found to have an effect as long as the task area was
properly covered in the field of view. For the particular task and
experimental setting, the optimal endoscope-to-target distance was
between 75 and 150 mm. Further research showed that the optical
axis-to-target view angle also has an influence on the task execution
in terms of execution time, applied force and error rate [20][21]. A

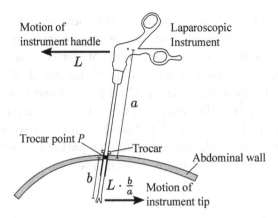

Figure 1.6: Illustration of the fulcrum effect in MIS. The motion scaling depends on the insertion depth, i.e. the relation between a and b.

correct rotational alignment of the endoscopic image on the monitor and the actual anatomical features is also favorable [22]. The results by Voorhost et al. [23] point in the same direction: It can be difficult to distinguish unwanted motions of the camera assistant from intended motions of the instruments, thereby hampering manipulation tasks.

Given these results, it is well known that the view quality provided in clinical practice is often not ideal [24]. Ideally, the camera assistant understands the procedure, is not affected by physical fatigue and can concentrate till the end of the intervention. In practice, camera assistants are often the most junior person in the OR and do not conform to any of these criteria. Shew et al. [25] note that "[...] it became apparent that there was much better utilization of the OR personnel. Prior to [the use of a laparoscope robot], nurses were the ones who were being asked to hold the camera and there was a great deal of dissatisfaction on their part with this task. This holds even more true in many academic settings where a medical student, perhaps the least trained or experienced camera holder available, is often asked to perform this extremely important task."

In summary, providing a suitable endoscopic view to the surgeon is important. The influence of endoscope positioning on surgical performance is well established based on objective task performance measures. Bad ergonomics in MIS could be improved, if space at the OR table can be freed up or the assistant is relieved from constantly holding the endoscope. The expected impact here is, as recently stated by Kassahun et al. [26] that "[e]ndowed with cognitive capabilities, surgical robots could take over the simpler parts of a task and allow surgeons to focus on the more crucial and complex parts of the procedure."

1.2 Medical Robotics

The major goal of research in the field of medical robotics is to adapt robotics technology for the medical domain. The vast majority of current robotics technology was developed in the context of industrial automation, where modern robotics originated in the late 1950s [27]. This does not only manifest itself in industrial robotics still being economically by far the most important sector, but also in the predominant technical choices. For manufacturing the primary concerns were to build robots with a high repeating accuracy, high speed and 24/7 availability. Tasks were and still are largely repetitive. The environment of the robots was designed to suit the tasks and robots. Every piece of handled equipment was by design fixed in a precisely known location. The robot's job was to perform exactly the same movements over and over. This sharply contrasts surgery, where variation in patient anatomy and even more in the clinical picture is the rule. Thus one of the main challenges in the field of medical robotics is preserving the advantages of classical robots, accuracy and endurance, but adapting to individualized and dynamic tasks. For more information on the history of robots in surgery see the overviews (newest first) by Kroh et al. [28], Pugin et al. [29], Kalan et al. [30] and Ewing et al. [31].

Another challenge is bringing together two very different fields of expertise. Each discipline does not only have its own domain of knowledge, but also very different notions for the same subject matter. A natural way to think about spatial relations for the roboticist are (Cartesian) coordinate systems and absolute units of measure. However, if these spatial relations address the human body, the anatomical vocabulary of surgeons is often much more adequate. The former vocabulary is based on what machines are good at and largely used for,[3] like precisely measuring angles and distances. The latter has always been intimately tied to educated human perception of complex shapes and structure. Still, precisely these different terminologies, which do not have direct correspondences in each other, must be translated back and forth in medical robotics (Fig. 1.7).

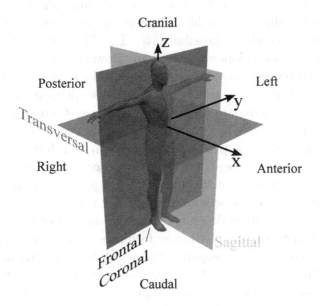

Figure 1.7: Anatomical terms of location and the patient coordinate system convention used throughout the thesis.

---

[3]Or at least, what machines have been good at and have been used for thus far.

As a first distinction medical robotics can be subdivided into telemanipulated and active robots [32]. Telemanipulated systems follow the master/slave model. In these systems, the surgeon does not physically interact with the patient, but uses an input device to control a robot that interacts with the patient. Apart from simple modifications of the input, such as scaling the motion or filtering out high-frequency low-amplitude motion (tremor), the robot performs exactly the motions as given by the surgeon. Since a human always remains in the loop, telemanipulation is very flexible, but at the same time a fully manual process. The da Vinci [33], Intuitive Surgical, is clinically by far the most widely used surgical robot. During interventions with the da Vinci, the surgeon sits at a surgical console that provides a stereo endoscopic view and controls the robot bimanually. Although clinical benefits could not be proven for abdominal surgery, teleoperation with the da Vinci might still prove benefitial where it renders laparoscopic procedures possible [34]. The MiroSurge system [35], DLR, is a bilateral teleoperation system. However, in contrast to the da Vinci, MiroSurge is not a commercial product and has no clinical approval. Yet, it is a relevant system because although strictly following the telemanipulation paradigm, it is a modular system made up of multiple independent light weight robots and it provides force feedback through its haptic input devices. In addition to these systems for telesurgery, most motorized endoscope holders in clinical use today, only offer manual control through joysticks, foot pedals or voice commands. These will be detailed in 2.1.

Active medical robots determine a significant part of their motions through algorithms. In its simplest form, the surgeon manually specifies a movement plan preoperatively, which is then intraoperatively executed by the robot. Following the suggestion by Moustris et al. [36], a robot that solely follows preprogrammed motions could be called an "automaton". The planning phase often takes place on medical imaging data, such as Computed tomography (CT) or Magnetic resonance imaging (MRI). Later on, at the beginning of the interven-

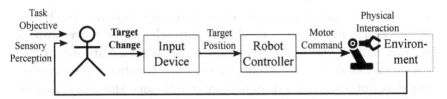

(a) Outline of a manually controlled robotic system. The robot only
moves while the operator issues new motion commands, otherwise
the robot is stationary.

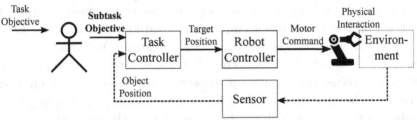

(b) Illustration of an active robot system. The external sensor feedback is optional and distinguishes between an "automaton" and an
"autonomous" robot.

Figure 1.8: Comparison of manual robot control (telemanipulation) and
active (autonomous) robot systems.

tion, the patient on the OR table must be registered[4] to the imaging
data and the robot. Once the registration has been performed, the
robot strictly follows the planned trajectory without further input
by the surgeon. ROBODOC [37], Integrated Surgical Systems, was
a clinically used robot working according to the described method.
The MAKO RIO robot [38], MAKO Surgical, combines elements from
telemanipulated and manually planned active robots. A preoperative
planning phase is combined with manual haptic control during the
intervention. While all robot movements remain under direct control
of the surgeon, he receives haptic feedback based on the preoperative
plan. The plan defines so called virtual fixtures, which create an

---

[4]Registration refers to the process of determining the geometric relationships
between two spatial reference systems. For further information, see 6.1.1.

artificial force that is opposite to the surgeon's movements. This is used to define areas where the burr is intended to be moved during the intervention and other areas that resist motions entering them.

A second kind of active robots makes intraoperative use of sensors[5] that determine or at least significantly influence the robot motion. Again, following [36], such a robot could be called "autonomous" because it performs actuation that is purposeful with respect to the environment. Many of these systems employ some kind of visual servoing (cf. 2.2.3) that closes the loop with the environment. Although a position controlled robot employees closed-loop control (Fig. 1.9a), only errors with respect to an internal reference, the target position, are compensated. With systems that use external sensors, such as visual servoing, the error with respect to a reference in the environment can be compensated (Fig. 1.9b). An example of an image guided robot in clinical use is the Cyberknife for radiotherapy [39].

A special issue in robotics for MIS is the trocar constraint (Fig. 1.10). The small incision in the patient's abdomen through which the trocars are inserted (Fig. 1.2) defines an invariant point of motion that must not be violated.[6] In particular, no lateral forces must be exerted to the trocar puncture site. Two degrees of freedom are constrained by the incision point on the surface of the abdomen. Thus, only four degrees of freedom are available. One consequence is that each point in the abdominal cavity can only be reached from one direction through each trocar. As will be seen in the following section, there are two principal approaches to observe the trocar constraint. The first approach employs standard – usually serial – kinematics as found in industrial robots. These would easily violate the trocar constraint under manual control in joint or Cartesian space. Therefore, the user is presented with an interface in spherical coordinates (cf. Fig. 2.4), which inherently obey the trocar constraint, with an optional rotation of the endoscope along its shaft. Often sensible maximum ranges of

---

[5]The basic shaft encoders required for position control of the individual robot joints are not considered here.

[6]Due to some flexibility of the abdominal wall, even when insufflated, the constraint is not a point in the strict sense.

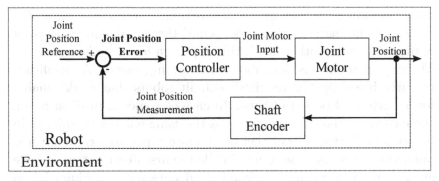

(a) A robot without external sensors: The closed-loop control can only
   compensate internal errors.

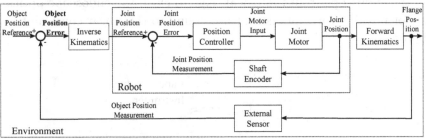

(b) A robot with an external sensor: The outer closed-loop control can
   also compensate errors with respect to an object reference in the
   environment.

Figure 1.9: Two kinds of closed-loop control in robotics.

motion are preset as an additional safety measure. The user input is
then mapped to joint values by means of the robot's regular inverse
kinematics. However, crucially, the interpolation is performed in the
spherical trocar space instead of joint or Cartesian space. The other
approach for maintaining the trocar constraint are special – often
parallel – kinematics that provide a remote center-of-motion in hardware. This has the advantage that the constraint is already built into
the robot's mechanics and is maintained independently of the control
software's correctness. After the initial manual positioning of the

robot, including the insertion of the instrument or endoscope into the trocar, all automatic motion is performed through the invariant point of motion. On the other hand, this approach has two disadvantages: The first is about custom robot hardware in general. A significant resource investment is required to built robots that work reliably for an extended period of time. In case of a special medical robot, these costs can not be spread across the same number of units as in industrial robotics. Thus either much more expensive or, even worse, unreliable robots are the result. While the first disadvantage is more an economical concern, the second disadvantage directly impedes on the robot's assistance function. For example, automatic withdrawal of the endoscope from the trocar, e.g. to clean the endoscope optics, is not possible with robots that are bound to the trocar constraint in hardware.

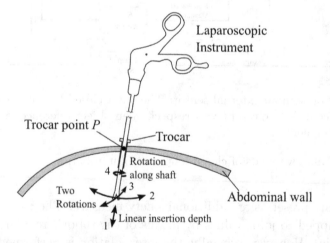

Figure 1.10: The figure illustrates the four available degrees of freedom for an instrument inserted into a trocar (1-4). The instrument must always pass through the invariant point of motion P. This requirement is referred to as trocar constraint.

Further information on the current state of medical robotics can be found in the comprehensive survey by Hoeckelmann et al. [40] and with a focus on commercial systems by Nakadete et al. [41].

1.3 Knowledge-based Cognitive Systems

All computer systems employ knowledge at least in the form of their software, which was written in order to fulfill a specific purpose. To this end, knowledge about how to proceed from a set of given inputs to the desired output was encoded into the computer program. However, in *knowledge-based systems* this knowledge does not only exist as executable program code, but also as an explicit model. A text file that documents and explains what knowledge was used for the creation of a certain program is not supposed to count here. Therefore, the explicit model is required to be meaningfully processable by a computer. For example, a natural language description of logical relations is not considered to fulfill this requirement. On the other hand, if the same relations are represented as a set of first order logic formulas with some well-defined syntax, the requirement is met. It is often helpful to distinguish between factual knowledge and learned know-how. Factual knowledge is commonly on a symbolic level, e.g. logic formulas, and can be directly expressed by an expert. Know-how is often subsymbolic and on the of level of data, e.g. parameters of differential equations. It must often be acquired by observation of an expert. To put both kinds in an example: A surgeon can write down details about the liver anatomy (factual knowledge) such as "The liver consists of two lobes. The gallbladder is attached to the right lobe." Yet, a surgeon, with any amount of surgical experience, cannot express how much force he applies during dissection to the liver lobe in objective units of measure – even though he does use the amount of force appropriate for the task (know-how).

Although there is no simple short definition, a *cognitive system* can be characterized by its abilities to

- perceive its environment,

- interpret this information,

- plan given the current situation to find means towards its objectives and

- purposefully act on the environment.

To ask whether a system is cognitive or not, poses the wrong question. The more appropriate question is to ask in which aspects is the system cognitive. The distinction is best illustrated by a few examples: A prime example of a system without any cognitive aspects is a pocket calculator.[7] An industrial robot would also not be considered to have any substantial cognitive aspects. It does exhibit some purposeful actuation even in case it always performs the same motion over and over because its position control is able to compensate some external influences on its movement. How narrow the cognition is can be seen when a work pieces that the robot is supposed to handle is missing: The robot will go through the exact same motions, even if 'empty-handed'. Moving along the dimension from non-cognitive to cognitive systems, a robot equipped with a camera to detect workpieces and put them into a box, shows more cognitive aspects. Relating to the previous example, if no workpiece is visible, the robot will simply not move since this would not add to its objective. Furthermore, the robot adapts better to changes in the environment, since even if a workpiece is not in the exact same location, the robot can recognize its position and move it. Yet, without further cognitive abilities, the robot would again not act purposefully in its environment when the unloading box is missing and continue to drop the parts on the floor. Looking at the very far end of the cognitive spectrum to a human handling parts, the size of the gap in dealing with different situations in which the objectives are still achieved becomes obvious.

The combination of knowledge-based systems and cognitive system is shown in Fig. 1.11. Following the paradigm of knowledge-based systems, the cognitive abilities are to a large part not encoded into

---

[7]Considering the buttons as environment perception and displaying of the result as action would render the whole intention behind the classification pointless.

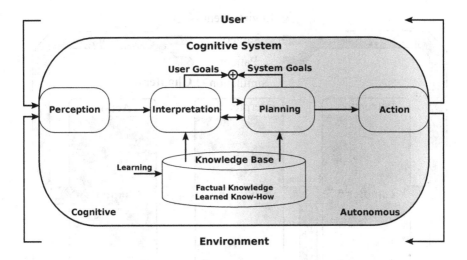

Figure 1.11: Block diagram of a knowledge-based cognitive system.

programs, but derived from explicit models of domain knowledge. Instead of separate programs for the perception of different objects, a more general object recognition component is implemented. Models of the relevant objects are read as additional input data by the recognition component. Similarly, planning in knowledge-based cognitive systems largely depends on a machine processable description of the task instead of being done by programs that contain the task hard-coded.

The individual concepts in Fig. 1.11 will be explained in detail and applied to automated camera guidance in chapter 3.

1.4 Overview of Thesis

The remainder of this thesis is organized as follows (cf. Fig. 1.12):

Chapter 2 first comprehensively surveys motorized endoscope holders in terms of their kinematics, manual control interfaces and study results. The second part of the chapter looks at different approaches to the automation of camera positioning and single-surgeon endoscope guidance. One direction of research adheres to fully manual

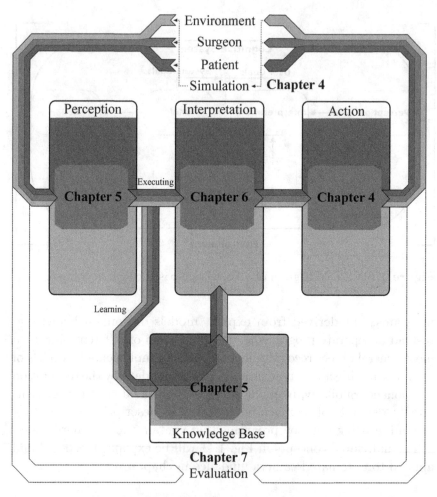

Figure 1.12: Structure of thesis. A survey of motorized endoscope robots and automated camera guidance is provided in chapter 2. The system architecture will be discussed in chapter 3.

control, while investigating alternative input modalities. The other important line of research looks into (semi-)automated camera control algorithms. The former aims at reducing the surgeon's additional cognitive burden for also having to control the camera. The goal of the latter is not to create a higher cognitive load in the first place by providing an automated camera positioner.

Chapter 3 provides an overview of the conceptual structure that underlies the knowledge-based endoscopic camera guidance system. Furthermore, the system architecture and design paradigm are explained. The main constituents of this structure are perception, interpretation, planning and action components together with a knowledge base of learned know-how and factual knowledge. These elements are first described in abstract terms and then put in relation with the specific task of creating an autonomous camera guidance.

In **chapter 4** the concrete hardware and software components that implement the knowledge-based system are introduced. It will be shown how all components are integrated into a modular research platform for robot-assisted minimally-invasive surgery. For this purpose, all sensors and actuators are represented as networked components with clearly defined interfaces. Different levels of abstraction in the interfaces facilitate interchangeability of (sub-)components, e.g. robot manipulators and endoscopic cameras. The individual software components are connected into a distributed computation graph through a soft real-time middleware. This modularity enabled evaluation of the endoscope control algorithms with different robots and in different environments. A simulation environment can transparently surrogate the hardware components, thereby enabling development outside the lab and more refined software engineering methods such as robot unit testing.

The topic of **chapter 5** is the perception, interpretation and learning pipeline required to build a camera guidance knowledge base. Recorded trajectories of the endoscope and surgical instruments during multiple interventions of a particular type make up the training set for the supervised machine learning pipeline. Labels are provided by experts as annotations of the suitability of the endoscopic view for a given situation. The result of the learning task is a camera guidance quality classifier, which serves as a model of adequate spatial relations between instruments and endoscope. Two particular challenges addressed here are, first, how to model spatial learning problems. Secondly, how to adapt the approach for the interdisciplinary field of surgical robotics, where only a few labeled data sets are available, which, in addition, often have a significant class imbalance.

Given the camera guidance quality classifier, **chapter 6** describes how it is used to realize a robot-based autonomous endoscope guidance – as a physical intraoperative assistance function. The endoscope guidance is implemented in the modular robot platform outlined above. The capabilities of the modular and networked platform architecture are utilized to implement the endoscope control algorithm on an abstract level. Whether instrument tips are extracted from the endoscope image or acquired through external marker-based systems and the robot kinematics that guide the endoscope, thus, become runtime details.

Having described the conceptual design, architecture, platform, learned knowledge base and intraoperative execution of the knowledge-based camera guidance system, **Chapter 7** details how the system was experimentally validated and its performance evaluated. The experimental setup is a series of laparoscopic surgical interventions, specifically rectal resection with total mesorectal resection, performed by surgeons in the OpenHELP phantom with camera assistance provided by a robot. Metrics for surgical task performance were employed in order to objectively asses the camera guidance quality and compare it to a human assistant. Facilitated by the modular implementation, the unmodified camera guidance component was evaluated with two widely different robots. It could be shown that the robot can learn from a human assistant as well as from a different robot. In addition, it was possible to further improve the guidance performance by using earlier robot-assisted interventions as training examples.

The final **chapter 8** concludes the work with a discussion of the advantages and drawbacks of the implemented system and its experimental performance. Additionally, pointers to ongoing and future research in the field of knowledge-based physical surgical assistance systems are provided.

2 Endoscope Robots and Automated Camera Guidance

2.1 A Survey of Motorized Endoscope Holders

This section describes in chronological order the development of motorized endoscope[1] holders. In the literature these are often referred to as active endoscope holders. However, this term is avoided here as it suggests active robots as defined in the previous chapter (p. 1.2) as opposed to telemanipulated robots. All endoscope holders treated in this section belong into the category of telemanipulated robots.

The focus in this section is on the mechanical structure and human-machine interfaces of the endoscope robots. A more in depth look at the approaches for the automation of camera guidance, is the topic of the following section (2.2). Given the short history of modern minimally-invasive surgery (cf. 1.1.1), the first attempts to replace the camera assistant with a robot have been quite early.

Before motorized endoscope holders, simple mechanical holders have been employed that must be unlocked, readjusted by hand and then relocked for each change in endoscope position. Examples of these mechanical holders are the Robotrac, Aesculap, the First Assistant, Loanard Medical Inc., the Omni-Tract, Minnesota Scientific and the Iron Intern, Automated Medical Products Corp. The system by Erbse et al. [42][43] is already a mechatronical system that uses piezoelectric actuators for locking and unlocking. A step beyond these devices originating in mechanical retracting systems for open surgery were

---

[1]Only rigid endoscopes that remain partially outside the patients body are included, e.g. laparoscopes. In particular this excludes flexible endoscopes, such as gastroscopes, and capsule endoscopes.

special kinematics with a built in remote center-of-motion.[2] One of these representatives is the TISKA Endoarm [44], which was developed at the Karlsruhe Research Center and commercialized by Karl Storz GmbH. TISKA is not purely mechanic, but uses electromagnetic friction to keep a position that is enabled and disabled by a foot pedal.

Although motorized, the Roboscope [45] is excluded from the survey because the only control mechanism it provides is manual hand guidance. In the same manner, modified endoscopes with panoramic optics augmented by motorized optical zoom and purely visual translation of the image, e.g. as presented by Kimura et al. [46] and the ImagTrac system [47], Olympus, are considered outside the intended scope. The Kaist Laparoscopic Assistant Robot (KaLAR) [48][49] that builds on a custom endoscope featuring an additional bending mechanism is therefore also excluded. The Robotic Flexible Laparoscope System (RFLS) [50] is controlled by head motion using a gyroscope, but since the control modality is very similar to the system in section 2.1.21 this flexible endoscope is not further elaborated. Tamadazte et al. [51] insert two additional miniature high-definition cameras with the endoscope into the trocar, thereby increasing the surgeon's field of view. The ViKY endoscope robot (cf. 2.1.9) is used to manually position the augmented endoscope, yet, further details about this system fall outside the scope set here.

Two crucial advantages of endoscope holders compared to a human assistant are a more stable image and the potential to take up less space around the operating table [17]. Even the fine motor tremor of the human camera assistant is reported to deteriorate the image stability [25].[3] Furthermore, the idea of solo surgery, i.e. performing laparoscopic procedures without human assistance, is a big motivational factor for many surgeons [52].

---

[2]Given the robot is positioned correctly, the mechanical structure of robot kinematics with a remote center-of-motion guarantee that the trocar constraint (Fig. 1.10) are maintained.

[3]See section 6.1.4 for a model and an empirical evaluation how vibrations influence robot-assisted endoscope guidance.

2.1.1 Endex

The Endex endoscopic positioning system [53], Andronic Devices Ltd., can be seen in the middle between mechanic endoscope holders and motorized ones (Fig. 2.1a). It only features a single actuated degree of freedom (Fig. 2.1b). Otherwise the Endex is a passive mechanical structure that is pneumatically locked and unlocked. The single motor uses the endoscope optics as a linear joint by means of a silicon roller. A foot pedal allows to move the orientationally fixed endoscope in and out of the trocar. The authors report their experience for using the Endex in over 60 gynecologic surgical procedures. Best user experience is reported for tasks that require an extended period of time in the same operative field. Spatial constraints are improved by attaching the holder to the other side of the OR table.

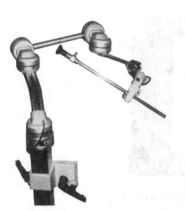

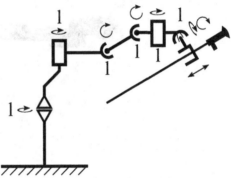

(a) Image of the Endex endoscope holder (Source: [53]).

(b) Endex kinematics: All passive joints l employ pneumatic locking, which is controlled with a release button. The endoscope is used as rail in the actuated linear joint.

Figure 2.1: The Endex endoscope holder.

2.1.2 AESOP (Automated Endoscope System for Optimal Positioning)

The Automated Endoscope System for Optimal Positioning (AESOP) was first described by Sackier and Wang [54] in 1994 (Fig. 2.2). A custom manipulator with 4 actuated and 2 passive joints is presented with a SCARA-like structure (Fig. 2.3). The AESOP joints are backdrivable, this feature is used to enable manual repositioning of the endoscope as with a mechanical holder. However, the surgeon has to pay attention to the robot's kinematic structure and must thus make sure to obey the trocar constraint by himself.[4] Other interfaces for manual control are pressure sensitive foot pedals and a joystick-like hand controller. The current endoscope position can also be stored and recalled later on.

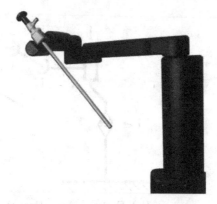

Figure 2.2: The AESOP endoscope holder (Source: [54]).

The AESOP, Computer Motion, was FDA-approved in 1994 [55] and subsequently evaluated in a number of clinical studies. Jacobs et al. show that using the foot pedal to control the robot leads to

---

[4]Employing the backdrivability with unpowered motors thus feels quite different than a robot that measures the external forces exerted by the surgeon and actively complies to them in task space instead of joint space. The latter is referred to as "hands-on" mode or "kinesthetic" mode. See the description of the LARS robot in the current section.

increased task completion times compared to manually guiding the endoscope [24]. In 1999 Arezzo et al. compared the duration and subjective rating of 70 laparoscopic experiments performed as solo surgery [52]. The original AESOP (AESOP 1000) controlled by foot pedals [56] and the later introduced voice-controlled AESOP 2000 [57] were compared with the passive TISKO Endoarm and human assistance. Human assistance had slightly, but significant, lower completion time compared to all other setups. Furthermore, it was found that although completion time with unmotorized endoscope holders was lower, the best subjective rating was given to the voice-controlled AESOP. Foot pedals and (finger-ring) joysticks were the least favorable control options, both in terms of duration and user experience. The authors note the relatively large space requirements of the AESOP and lack of support for 30 degree optics. The former is largely due to the large cart the AESOP is attached to and not the robot arm.

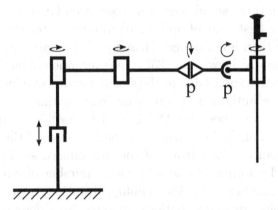

Figure 2.3: Kinematics of the AESOP endoscope holder. Joints marked with a letter p are unactuated passive joints.

For urological interventions Partin et al. [58] report results from 17 procedures performed with AESOP assistance. No increase in operating time compared to human assistance was found. However, in three cases intraoperative bleeding occurred and required human camera assistance. For gynecological surgery Mettler et al. [59] describe their experience with the voice-controlled AESOP. Although the AESOP provides a more stable image and results in reduced operative times, at the same time "the whole procedure requires more concentration from the surgeon". Kavoussi et al. reports a significantly steadier endoscopic image and no difference in operative times with robotic assistance [60]. Ballantyne reports similar results with respect to image stability and operating time in solo surgery of laparoscopic colectomies [55].

The newer AESOP 3000 was evaluated by Nebot et al. [61] in a phantom box and compared to the EndoAssist with head-tracking as input modality (cf. p. 35 in this section). Even with the improved speech recognition of the newer AESOP, the authors report frequent voice recognition errors that adversely affect the surgeon's performance. Punt et al. [62] evaluate control of endoscope zoom and light intensity through voice commands, a touch panel and a human assistant. Although there are also several recognition failures, voice control is deemed the best control option. Kipfmüller notes that use of the AESOP results in less frequent cleaning of the optics [63]. Another aspect reported by Shew et al. [25] is the prevention of motion sickness in small operative spaces due to the steadier endoscope image. On the other hand, the authors note a relevant learning time for the surgeon. For thoracic sympathectomy (VATS) for hyperhidrosis procedures[5] Martins Rua et al. [64] compared the performance of the AESOP to human assistance. Each group of the randomized study comprised 19 patients. Performance endpoints were number of wrong camera movements, number of optics cleaning, duration of procedure and several endpoints related to patient outcome. No difference was found in the patient endpoints and camera movements. The optics had to be cleaned less often, on average 0.22 to 0.42, but operation time was longer with an average of 12.89 to 9.89 minutes. In a study of 11 AESOP-assisted and 15 human-assisted colectomies, Merola et

---

[5]Clamping or dividing the sympathetic nerves inside the chest to cure abnormally increased sweating.

al. [65] find that neither length of operation nor patient outcome are significantly different. At the same time the robot reduced the number of required OR staff. The preference of some surgeons for robot assistance is believed to stem from "a subjective sense of better control of their surgical field contributes to this preference. The fluid movement of the robotic camera holder reduces motion sickness, eliminates the wandering of the laparoscope caused by an inattentive human assistant, keeps the picture still and steady until the surgeon commands it to move, and prevents inadvertent rotation of the laparoscope." Proske et al. [66] find no difference in terms of complications, duration of procedure or hospitalization between human-assisted and robot-assisted cholecystectomies and colectomies. The study group included 47 patients operated a year earlier with a human assistant and 50 patients operated with AESOP assistance.

Despite these positive results, there are also known general limitations of the AESOP [55]:

- Control of the camera robot with voice or joysticks is slow compared to human assistance for rapid changes of the visual field.

- Voice control can distract other OR staff.

- Manual control encourages settling for a single visual field instead of going back and forth between better suited ones.

Kraft et al. [67] compared the AESOP to human assistance for laparoscopic cholecystectomy and hernioplasty in a randomized study with two groups of 120 patients. For cholecystectomy, they found that the preoperative setup time was 5 minutes longer in case of robotic assistance. Also the operating time was about 5 minutes longer than with a human assistant for a median overall time of 30 minutes. Unsurprisingly, the voice-controlled AESOP required many more explicit commands than the human assistant. On a scale from 1 to 5 the subjective evaluation of the AESOP was 0.6 lower and the ability to achieve optimal focus was also worse by 0.6 points. However, the authors note that the human assistants in the control group were remarkably well trained with an average of 100 past assistances.

The AESOP is also part of the ZEUS telemanipulation robot described later in this section (p. 69).

2.1.3 Begin and Hurteau et al.

Begin and Hurteau et al. [68][69] presented a robotic camera holder in 1995.[6]. The system used a small industrial robot (CRS A460) with six degrees of freedom (DoF). An additional passive universal joint was used to fix the endoscope to the robot flange (Fig.2.5). Positioning of the endoscope was performed manually by the surgeon by means of a simple joystick. The joystick input was mapped to spherical coordinates centered around the camera trocar (Fig. 2.4). Thereby, the surgeon directly controlled the altitude (left-right motion), zenith (up-down motion) and radius (zoom motion). After an animal study, the system was evaluated in eight patients. It was shown that the surgeon was able to complete all procedures without a human camera assistant.

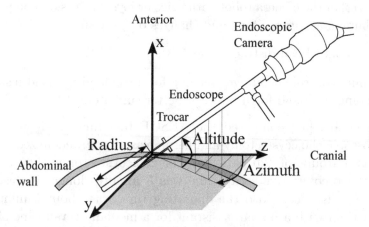

Figure 2.4: Illustration of a spherical coordinate system centered around the endoscope trocar.

---

[6]The first human applications and the paper submission were even two years earlier in 1993 [70]

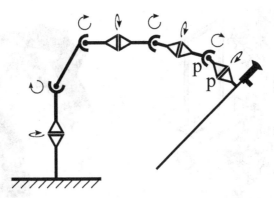

Figure 2.5: Kinematics of the CRS A460 together with a passive universal joint as used in the system by Begin et al.

2.1.4 LARS (Laparoscopic Assistant Robot System) / PLRCM (Parallel-Linkage Remote-Center-of-Motion)

The LARS [71] or PLRCM [72] robot[7] was published in 1995 by Taylor and Funda et al. (Fig. 2.6). It features a custom robot manipulator with a remote center-of-motion defined through four bar linkage kinematics serially coupled with a 3-axis linear cartesian stage (Fig.2.7). As a result, the trocar constraint is already taken care for in hardware. This improves patient safety by largely prohibiting injuries of the abdominal wall through unintended robot movements. A force-torque sensor mounted at the manipulator flange provides additional safety by monitoring the forces exerted by the robot. However, friction in the trocar and the necessary deformation of tissue does not allow highly sensitive force thresholds.

LARS implements two different human-machine interfaces for manual control. The first is an instrument mounted joystick that is basically directly mapped to the robot's rotational degrees of freedom (DoF). Alternatively, the robot can be controlled by directly exerting additional forces on the endoscope. These external forces are measured by

---

[7]The name LARS will be used for both publications.

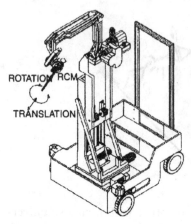

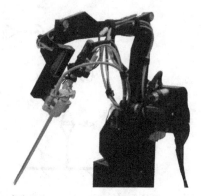

(a) Schematic drawing of LARS (Source: [71]).

(b) Upper part of the LARS endoscope holder (Source: [73]).

Figure 2.6: The LARS / PLRCM endoscope positioner.

the force-torque sensor and the robot complies with them by moving along the force vector, i.e. "hands-on". This cannot be used at the same time as the described safety feature based on the force-torque sensor. Furthermore, the authors consider adding speech commands as a option for direct control. Beyond the manual control modes, LARS also comprises a less direct control modality: The surgeon can use the joystick to move a superimposed cursor on the endoscopic display. He thereby selects an anatomical feature in the image that the endoscope is supposed to put in the center of the field of view. In order to map the two-dimensional monitor selection of the surgeon to a 3D point inside the patient triangulation is used. If a stereo endoscope is in use[8] this can be accomplished from the two camera perspectives. In case of a monoscopic laparoscope the robot slightly displaces it in order to acquire the two required images. Once the target point is known, the robot moves the endoscope in order to center on the target. LARS was in-vivo evaluated on pigs in 1994.

---

[8]Stereo laparoscopes were not available at the time.

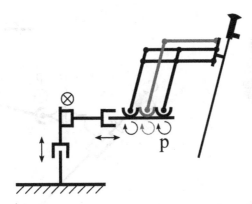

Figure 2.7: Kinematics of the Laparoscopic Assistant Robot System
(LARS). The structure of the two parallel linkages is shown
simplified. Passive joints are marked by p.

In a later publication [73], optimal control of the robot under trocar
constraint (cf. Fig. 1.10) is formulated as an optimization problem.
This enables a generic description of task-dependent control modes
including motion constraints. The control approach is compatible
with kinematically deficient systems, i.e. having less than 6 degrees of
freedom, as well as kinematically redundant systems, i.e. more than
6 DoFs. An example of the former is the LARS with 5 DoF and an
example of the later is the HISAR with 7 DoF (see 2.1.5).

2.1.5 HISAR (Hopkins-IBM Surgical Assistant Robot)

Funda et al. [74] report on application of the Hopkins-IBM Surgical
Assistant Robot (HISAR) as endoscope holder (Fig. 2.8a). HISAR is
ceiling-mounted and features 7 degrees of freedom (Fig. 2.8b). Two of
these degrees are passive. One of these DoFs is the actuated rotation
of the camera around the endoscope optics. Therefore four actuated
DoFs are used for positioning the optics' eye piece and thereby the
spherical orientation, insertion depth and rotation along the endoscope
shaft.

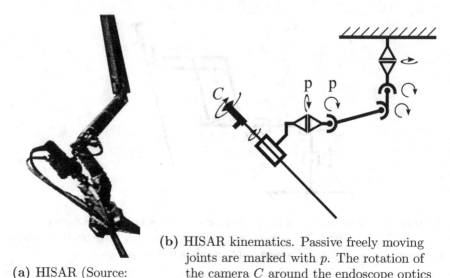

(b) HISAR kinematics. Passive freely moving
joints are marked with p. The rotation of
(a) HISAR (Source: the camera C around the endoscope optics
[72]).   is also motorized.

Figure 2.8: The Hopkins-IBM Surgical Assistant Robot (HISAR).

A comparison of the LARS/PLRCM with the HISAR with respect to safety, ergonomics and control are presented by the same authors [72]. They find that there are trade-offs to be made between these criteria. Main differences relate to precision of motion, especially under external disturbances, robot workspace and the space required by the robot in the OR. In case of the robots under comparison, the LARS is more precise, but with a much smaller working volume and it blocks a lot more relevant space in the OR. For safety reasons, the ability to measure force-torque with LARS due to the fully constrained endoscope is beneficial. On the other hand the backdrivability of the HISAR can also be seen as a safety feature in case of electronic failures.

Funda et al. conclude their evaluation with valuable insights into robotic assistance for surgery: "It is difficult to design a general purpose surgical robot. The workspace, ergonomic and precision requirements associated with different procedures vary greatly. Once a promising class of applications for robots in surgery is identified, a specific mechanism and design approach may be required to adequately address the application requirements within cost constraints. However, the manipulator itself is only one part of an overall system which includes control electronics, computers and software, human-machine interfaces, surgical end-effectors, and much more."

2.1.6 Laparobot, EndoSista, EndoAssist

In course of the development of the EndoAssist, Armstrong Healthcare Ltd., the intermediate prototype systems were known as Laparobot and for a longer period of time as EndoSista [75]. The EndoAssist was then introduced as a commercial product in 1998 [76]. For the sake of brevity and given their minor differences, only the kinematics of the final EndoAssist are described. The EndoAssist is not attached to the OR table, but is integrated into a wheeled cart that is positioned around the OR table. With its high vertical axis and long central boom, EndoAssist is intended to be placed behind the surgeon and to reach over him. The actuated kinematics are made up of the vertical axis and two rotational degrees of freedom at the end of the overhead boom (Fig. 2.10). A remote center-of-motion is implemented by an additional offset linkage that connects to the endoscope [75]. Proper positioning of the EndoAssist with respect to the camera trocar is facilitated by two lasers in the overhead boom.

A very relevant feature of the EndoAssist in this survey relates to its unconventional control interface. The EndoAssist uses head-tracking together with a simple foot switch [78]. The surgeon wears a headband that contains electromagnetic transmitters which provide the relative movement to an receiver mounted at the endoscopic monitor. In order to allow free head movement and to prevent unintended movement of the endoscope, a foot switch is used to engage control over the robot movement. If the surgeon wants the endoscope to move left, he presses the foot switch and turns his head slightly left. The robot will move into this direction until the surgeon turns his head into another direction or disengages the robot by releasing the foot switch. This is quite different from the approach of directly linking head

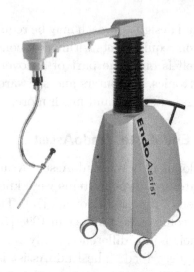

Figure 2.9: The EndoAssist endoscope holder (Source: [77]).

motion to motion of the endoscope. For example, Voorhost et al. [79] performed experiments on directly linking endoscopic perspective and head rotation of the surgeon. Although this research has been resumed recently [80], the relationship between instruments and position of the surgeon poses many obstacles in practice.

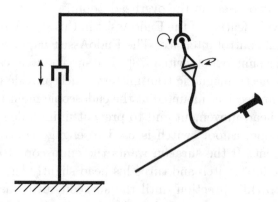

Figure 2.10: Kinematics of the EndoAssist endoscope holder.

The first clinical trials of the prototype system were conducted in 1993 [81]. A major benefit of the system, as reported by Finlay [82], the founder of Armstrong Healthcare Ltd., compared to human assistant is the steady image - especially at the end of long procedures. Aiono et al. [78][83] report results of a randomized clinical study with 96 laparoscopic cholecystectomies conducted by six surgeons. About half of the interventions were performed with robot assistance and the other half with human assistance. In their results mean operating time with robotic assistance was 8 minutes shorter for an average duration of 70 minutes. Furthermore, they found a smaller variation in the operating time. Only three interventions were required to fully master the learning curve for head control. Regarding trainees, Aiono et al. see a benefit in freeing them from camera work and thus allowing them to focus more on relevant matters. Yet, they acknowledge the concern of junior team members not taking part in robot-assisted procedures anymore in the future. In the domain of urological surgery, Kommu et al. [77][84] report the results of a clinical study with 51 procedures, half of which are performed robot-assisted. The evaluated endpoints were: body part discomfort score (BPDS), subjective usability, number of required lens cleanings, setup time, overall operative time, subjective surgical performance and number of required rearrangements of the EndoAssist. Although all procedures could be performed with the EndoAssist, in several occasions the arm had to be relocated. In general more frequent lens cleaning was required in the robot-assisted case. BPDS scores were equal for both assistances. Depending on the procedure type, usability was equal or lower to human assistance. No difference was found in setup time and surgical performance.

Yavuz et al. [85] compare the performance of the AESOP and the EndoSista (EndoAssist) for standard camera tasks in training boxes. Their results show a much better performance in terms of task duration for preprogrammed movements (position memory) with the AESOP. Furthermore, voice control of the AESOP was found to be superior to head control in the EndoSista. Yet, the results must be taken with caution since all experiments were performed by a single operator.

Qualitatively, the authors note that the AESOP feels less bulky and quality of voice control is diminished in noisy environments. Wagner et al. [86] also compare AESOP to EndoAssist. However, their results are from two groups of 20 patients each undergoing laparoscopic radical prostatectomy (LRP)[9] with assistance by AESOP or EndoAssist. EndoAssist was controlled by the surgeon through the head motion interface. AESOP was controlled by an experienced assistant. Average setup time of AESOP was lower, 2 minutes, compared to EndoAssist, 5.3 minutes. Only in 1 out of 11 steps in the intervention was a significant difference between assistant-controlled AESOP and surgeon-controlled EndoAssist, which favored the EndoAssist. Even though an assistant is required for LRP, the procedure subjectively benefited from robot assistance because the assistant could fully focus on his other tasks. Nebot et al. [61] performed a similar study in which they evaluate the EndoAssist and AESOP 3000 performance for complex camera tasks in box trainers. They find the head-tracking controlled EndoAssist to be significantly faster than the voice controlled AESOP. A large part of the result is attributed to the continuous control of the EndoAssist compared to the discrete step-wise control of the AESOP. However, better usability is ascribed to the AESOP voice control, given the complexity of precise head movements together with the requirement to press a foot switch. Den Boer et al. [87] compare AESOP to a passive endoscope holder (PASSIST) and to human assistance. From 78 laparoscopic cholecystectomies 30 were performed as solo surgery. Operative times were not significantly different with 42 to 49 minutes average for assisted surgery compared to solo surgery. The number of endoscope repositioning was with an average of 49 times much lower with AESOP than the 114 times with human assistance.

2.1.7 FIPS Endoarm

The FIPS Endoarm [88] is a remote controlled endoscope positioning arm developed by the Karlsruhe Research Center (FZK) and the

---

[9]Surgical removal of the whole prostate gland.

University of Tuebingen. FIPS was later brought to market by Karl Storz GmbH.

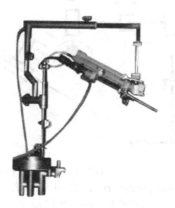

Figure 2.11: The FIPS Endoarm (Source: [88]).

Over 300 phantom procedures were performed without human assistance. The authors report shorter operative times compared to human assistance. However, even shorter times are reported for assistance by a passive endoscope holder (TISKA Endoarm, cf. p. 24). They conclude that "none of the solutions tested showed an intuitiveness and reliability competitive with hand positioning". Furthermore, the findings suggest best overall ergonomics when the endoscope robot is placed on the opposite side of the OR table. The FIPS Endoarm was later used as part of the ARTEMIS teleoperation system [89] for MIS. A version of FIPS was also experimentally used for gynecological laser laparoscopy [90].

Buess et al. [91] report about a randomized study involving phantom experiments of laparoscopic cholecystectomy. Three groups of 15 interventions each were performed: human assisted, assistance by FIPS Endoarm controlled with the finger-joystick and voice-controlled FIPS Endoarm assistance. Although the joystick interface was judged more intuitive, intervention times were slightly lower with voice control. One major disadvantage in the voice command interface was found to be the limited motion of each command. For example, a long move

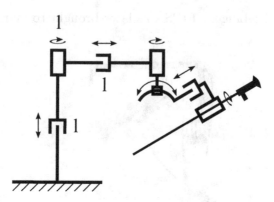

Figure 2.12: Kinematics of the FIPS Endoarm. Unactuated mechanically locked joints are marked with l. The remote center-of-
motion is realized through a C-arch mechanism.

into the same direction requires a sequence of multiple identical voice
commands. While the intervention time with the FIPS Endoarm was
lower than with human assistance, the overall time including setup
and break-down was significantly longer. Yet, the systems allows
to reduce the number of required assistants [92]. Arezzo et al. [93]
attests FIPS the best results and most intuitive user experience in a
series of 400 phantom cholecystectomies in comparison with AESOP
and EndoAssist.

A later iteration of the FIPS Endoarm, named FELIX, featured
visual tracking of instruments [94]. The image was divided into three
areas, central, inner and outer region, if the instrument leaves the
inner region the endoscope moves towards it until it is within this
region again.

2.1.8 Munoz et al., ERM (Endoscopic Robotic Manipulator)

The setup presented by Munoz et al. [95] in 2000 consists of a Stäubli
RX60 with two passive rotational DoFs in the endoscope adapter.
This kinematic structure is identical to the one in Begin et al. (see

Fig. 2.5). A mapping of Cartesian to spherical coordinates is employed for control (cf. Fig. 2.4). Voice-control with discrete commands and joystick with four degrees of freedom, modelled after an endoscope, is used to control the endoscope in spherical coordinates with the camera trocar as center of motion. Several phantom and pig experiments were conducted with the system to show its general feasibility [96].

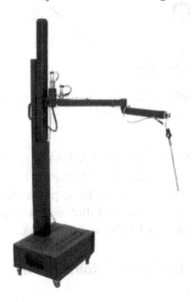

Figure 2.13: The ERM endoscope holder (Source: [97]).

In 2001 Munoz et al. [98] present new custom kinematics, later called ERM, for an endoscope holder (Fig. 2.13). The new SCARA-like robot (Fig. 2.14) features one linear and two actuated rotational joints together with two passive rotational joints at the endoscope holder. An extensive discussion of the required workspaces and possible kinematics solutions can be found in a later publication [97]. Voice control and remote control via a 3D mouse, SpaceBall, provide manual control over the endoscope movement [99].

In 2005 a follow up publication describes a refined version of the ERM (Fig. 2.14) together with in vivo and clinical results [100]. A

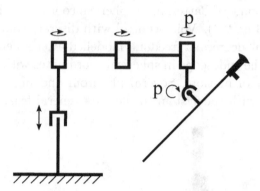

Figure 2.14: Kinematics of the custom endoscope arm (ERM) described by Munoz et al. in 2001.

failure mode and effects analysis (FMEA) is undertaken to identify possible failure szenarios and their potential hazard for the patient. Munoz et al. [101] report that in the experiments with 16 patients the robot performance was good. Robot-assisted operating times were shorter and the optics had to cleaned less often.

2.1.9 LER (Light Endoscope Robot), ViKY (Vision Kontrol endoscopY)

The Light Endoscope Robot (LER) was introduced by Berkelman et al. in 2002 [102]. From the onset the goal was to develop a much smaller and lighter endoscope manipulator compared to all previous systems. The very first design was a cable driven robot actuated by pneumatic artifical muscles actuators. An immediately following update of this design replaced the pneumatic actuators by electric motors for their higher accuracy and easier control [103]. Already the next prototype of 2003 [104] was then very similar to what became a commercial product under the name ViKY later on. Therefore the first design will not be discussed here. The kinematic diagram of LER is shown in Fig. 2.15. Two passive universal joints together with a passive rotational joint that can be mechanically locked in unison position the actuated part of the LER concentrically around the camera trocar (Fig. 2.16a). The actuated part consists of a special serial kinematic: A round rack and pinion actuator, a C-arch mechanism and a linear rack and pinion actuator that clips to the endoscope. This structure implements spherical kinematics directly in hardware. Each 'natural' movement (left ↔ right, up ↔ down and in ↔ out) is directly mapped to a single actuated joint. Given a horizontal attachment, the image horizon remains stable. Since no rotation around the endoscope shaft is possible, LER is only suitable for 0° optics. Both passive and actuated part – including gears and the brushless motors – can be autoclave sterilized and thus no part of the robot requires draping. Each joint is backdrivable if the motors are switched off. This can be used for initial positioning. Basic manual control interfaces are a miniature keypad that is clipped to the instrument handle and voice commands. Long et al. [105][106] reports on an initial pig and cadaver experiment series undertaken from 2003 to 2005 with the LER. The compactness of the LER and easy setup is reported as a practical advantage. After initial breakdowns of the hardware, the later prototypes proved sufficiently reliable.

The LER was commercialized after clinical studies (2007) with FDA approval in 2008 under the name ViKY (Vision Kontrol endoscopY) [107]. A multidirectional foot pedal and voice commands via bluetooth headsets are provided as control interfaces (Fig. 2.16b). In addition, the current endoscope pose can be saved and later on recalled by voice commands. According to Gumps et al. [108] setup time of the ViKY is significantly shorter compared to AESOP, on average 41 to 253 seconds. The authors report a similar time reduction in (simulated) emergency removal, 3 seconds for ViKY and 8 seconds for AESOP. Voice control is evaluated to have a low success rate of 71%[10] and thus the foot pedal was judged superior. Although the ViKY is much more compact with respect to space at the OR table, the relatively large footprint of the rack and pinion disk can be obstructive for the instrument trocars. The initial clinical study

---

[10]The authors report 67% for AESOP 3000.

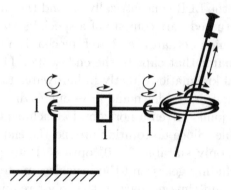

Figure 2.15: Kinematics of the LER and ViKY endoscope holders. An
important difference in kinematics between LER and ViKY
is the realization of the linear axis: LER uses a cable-driven
design counteracted by a compression spring. ViKY employs a rack and pinion actuator. The first three joints l
are mechanically locked.

comprised 53 patients with prolapse surgeries, prostatectomies[11] and
cholecystectomies being the dominant procedures. Unfortunately, no
comparative data to human assisted interventions is provided for the
reported robot-assisted operative times. The setup time for ViKY
was found to be around 5 minutes. As main advantage the freeing of
one assistant's hand is noted, lack of amplitude of motion as main
limitation.

Long et al. [109] present a study of 20 patients undergoing urologic
surgery with ViKY assistance. One patient withdrew his consent for
robotic-assistance. In two cases the robot could not be used: Once
due to malfunction and in the other case due to difficult adhesiolysis[12].
Out of 17 interventions started with ViKY assistance, 5 were not
completed with the robot. In one case the voice control failed and in
four cases the surgical conditions required human assistance. Complete
autonomy of the surgeon over the camera is stated as main surgical

---

[11]Surgical removal of the prostate gland.
[12]Surgical devision of irregular adhesions.

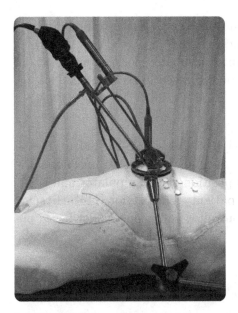

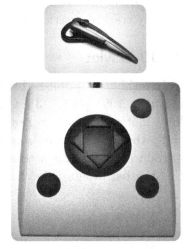

(a) The ViKY endoscope holder attached to the OR table and centered around the trocar of a medical phantom.

(b) ViKY control interfaces: Discrete voice commands and a foot pedal for continues control

Figure 2.16: The ViKY endoscope holder.

advantage. Limitations in the motion range of ViKY were found to represent a practical issue. Furthermore, the robot becomes less usable, if a lot or very wide motions are required. The authors qualify the results by stating that "a pilot study that can only assess the feasibility and the safety of the procedures using the robot. Further studies should investigate the clinical impact."

In 2009 Berkelman et al. [110][111] presented a telemanipulation setup for MIS based on the kinematics of the ViKY system. It consists of three ViKY robots, two small ones for the instruments[13] and a middle sized one for the endoscope, together with a master console

---

[13]Custom instruments with an actuated wrist are used in the setup.

featuring two haptic devices, Phantom Omni. Voice commands are used to control the endoscope guiding ViKY.

Research by Voros et al. [107] into automated positioning based on visually tracked instruments will be discussed in section 2.2.

2.1.10 Naviot

Kobayashi et al. published the design of a novel five-bar linkage mechanism in 1998 [112][113]. One particular goal was to mechanically limit motion to a safe region and position the manipulator and especially the motors away from the patient. The Naviot [114], Hitachi, introduced in 2003, is a remote-controlled endoscope holder based on this five-bar design (Fig. 2.17).

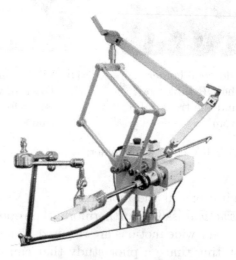

Figure 2.17: The Naviot endoscope holder (Source: [115]).

The five-bar linkage mechanism (Fig. 2.18) mechanically limits the range of motion to 45° horizontally and 25° vertically. Insertion depth is fixed, instead a motorized optical zoom is employed. A two button controller that is attached to the laparoscopic instrument is used to control endoscope orientation and optical zoom.

The system was initially evaluated through seven cholecystectomies in 2002, which showed the feasibility of the mechanism and its control. A later study by Tanoue et al. [115] compared a group of ten cholecystectomies with Naviot assistance to human assistance. The average total operative time of 89.3 minutes with the Naviot assistance was found to be significantly longer compared to human-assisted interventions with an average of 74.8 minutes. This additional time was largely due to the Naviot setup time. Using a shorter endoscope in combination with an optical zoom is reported to be beneficial because of less chance for contact with organs.

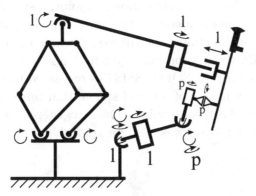

Figure 2.18: Kinematics of the Naviot. The endoscope can only be rotated in two dimensions. Zoom is achieved by optical means. The lower passive kinematic chain fixes the endoscope's center of motion. Intraoperative locked joints l and free moving passive joints p are marked.

Yoshino et al. [116] evaluated the Naviot robot in two patients for thoracoscopic surgery[14]. Although the experiments were successful, concerns are raised about usability of the Naviot for more complex procedures given its small motion range. Yamada et al. [117] also successfully tested the Naviot in two thoracoscopic interventions.

---

[14]VATS: Video-assisted thoracoscopic surgery

2.1.11 SOLOASSIST

The SOLOASSIST [118], AKTORmed GmbH, was introduced as endoscope holder for visceral, urological and gynecological surgery. The SOLOASSIST directly clamps to the OR table. It consists of three actuated rotational and two passive rotational joints (Fig. 2.20). All actuated joints are fluidic actuators with integrated track measurements. By means of an overpressure function, each joint is backdrivable with a defined force. The camera end of the endoscope is positioned in three translational dimensions around the camera trocar. Because the endoscope tip is situated inside the trocar and the rotational freedom provided by the passive universal joint, a spherical motion around the trocar point results (cf. Fig. 1.10). In order to allow natural movement directions, the surgeon controls the robot not by translation in a Cartesian coordinate system, but in a spherical one (cf. Fig. 2.4). To this end, the SOLOASSIST is registered to the trocar in the setup phase by means of a metal sphere that must be manually positioned above the trocar point. Once registered, a sterilizable instrument-mounted joystick is used for control.

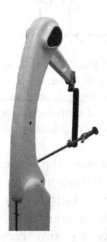

Figure 2.19: The SOLOASSIST endoscope holder (Source: [119]).

Gillen et al. [120] compared the performance of SOLOASSIST to a human camera assistant for cholecystectomies in two groups of 63 respectively 60 patients. Three experienced surgeons performed a total of 123 procedures. A majority of 47 out of 63 robot assisted operations were performed by a surgeon having a lot of experience working with the SOLOASSIST. Human assistance was provided by well experienced residents. The authors found that total operation time was significantly lower for the human-assisted group with an average of 90 to 104 minutes. However, the OR staff minutes, identical for solo surgery using SOLOASSIST, but twice the amount in case of human assistance, strongly favor robotic assistance with 104 to 180 minutes. The authors report that 4.8% of the procedures started with robotic assistance required a switch to human assistance. In these three cases intraoperative complications occurred. The three surgeons assigned the SOLOASSIST an average of 2 on a scale of 1 to 5 for the attributes handling, required force, quality of camera view and general satisfaction with the system. About two uncontrolled or unexpected camera movements per operation were registered. For laparoscopic surgery Holländer et al. [121] report on 1033 procedures performed with SOLOASSIST. In summary eight of the nine surgeons interviewed about their experience preferred robotic over human assistance because of better image stability and control over their view. In 71 cases the robot had to be removed and replaced by a human assistant.

For gynecological surgery Beckmeier et al. [122] evaluated the SOLOASSIST in 104 patients. The SOLOASSIST was used with conventional 2D endoscopes for the first 63 patients and then replaced by the Einstein Vision system, Aesculap / B. Braun Melsungen AG. The latter uses a slightly modified SOLOASSIST as camera holder together with a 3D endoscope. For the purpose of this endoscope holder overview, both systems can be treated jointly. Setup time averaged 7 minutes, the learning curve is reported to be about 20 cases. Total operative time with robot assistance increased by 4 minutes from 110 to 114 minutes. Handling was evaluated with a score 2 (good) on a scale from 1 to 5. An average of 1 unwanted

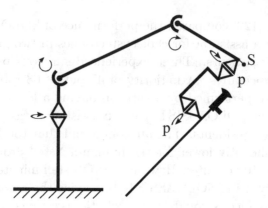

Figure 2.20: Kinematics of the SOLOASSIST. The sphere S at the end
of the second link is used for registration with the pivot
point. The two joints p close to the endoscope are free
moving passive ones.

camera movement per operation was recorded. Furthermore, the
authors stress the economic advantage of not requiring a camera
assistant.

In the area of head and neck surgery Kristin et al. [123] evaluated
and adapted SOLOASSIST as a motorized camera holder. Starting
with feasibility evaluations of the SOLOASSIST for interventions in
nose, nasopharynx[15] and larynx[16] conducted in anatomical specimens,
it was found that the unmodified robot was not well suited. Points that
severely hindered the application were: Too high movement speed, not
adjustable motion speed and lack of force sensing and force feedback.
Especially the latter threatens patient safety because of potential
tissue perforations. In summary, the much tighter spaces around the
endoscope in head and neck surgery compared to visceral surgery make
robots such as the SOLOASSIST unfit for them. A first modification
replaced the endoscope adapter by a quick release fastener, such as
a magnetic connector, for faster removal of the endoscope from the

---

[15]Part of the upper respiratory system between mouth and nasal cavity.
[16]The voice box.

surgical area. In a later publication [124] measurements of forces that occur during sinus surgery were undertaken. Computer-aided design (CAD) was used to evaluate different adapted kinematics for head and neck surgery. Although prototypes were built, no detailed results are provided. Furthermore, the interoperative movements of a hand-held endoscope in head and neck interventions were recorded and analysed [119]. The maximum motions, volumes and enveloping bodies were calculated on a total of 27 sinus, 30 mastoid cavity and 14 larynx endoscopies. Based on these findings in the ENT[17] area, modifications of the SOLOASSIST were proposed. Foremost, the authors state that the "endoscope holder needs five degrees of freedom for use in head and neck surgery instead of only three degrees of freedom (as in abdominal surgery)."

In his MD thesis[18] from 2014, Maifeld [125] evaluates the SO-LOASSIST with respect to: Emergency conversion to open surgery; Performance in phantom tasks; In vivo performance on pigs with special attention to the reachability of all abdominal quadrants; and comparison of SOLOASSIST to AESOP and manual camera guidance in phantoms with respect to trajectory stability. Maifeld also poses the question why after more than 30 years of motorized endoscope holders, no system has gained wide clinical acceptance. In the experiments SOLOASSIST had a longer setup time, 297 seconds, compared to the AESOP, 129 seconds. Yet, both times are much shorter than the average preparation time for laparoscopic cholecystectomy of 22.2 minutes [126]. Further results are the mean task time of 7.7 minutes for SOLOASSIST compared to 4.5 minutes for AESOP. It was also more difficult to exactly follow a predefined trajectory with the SO-LOASSIST. Subjective evaluation of intuitive use and cognitive load also favored AESOP. In contrast, stability of the horizon was judged to be superior for the SOLOASSIST. Concerns are raised about tension on camera cable and light cable that can build up undetected during the course of an intervention. Qualitatively, the delay between press

---

[17]Ear, Nose and Throat.
[18]The thesis is written in German.

of the joystick buttons and movement of the robot was found to be too long. Control of the robot was found to be difficult close to the trocar point. The latter is likely due to the singularities that occur close to the trocar point when mapping from Cartesian to spherical coordinates (cf. 5.3.2 and 6.1.5). The author reports from a series of twelve cholecystectomies on pigs that operative time was about equal to human assistance. The surgeons preferred the SOLOASSIST in these experiments because of a reduction in corrective camera motions. Even though in some parts of the intervention, the surgeon and SOLOASSIST impeded each other in their workspace. Part of the thesis is also an acceptance survey based on the answers of 25 surgeons. 76% have no experience with robotic assistance systems, yet, 88% regard mechatronic support systems as desirable.

2.1.12 LapMan

The LapMan endoscope manipulator (Fig. 2.21), Medsys, introduced in 2004 [127], is primarily used in gynecological surgery. The LapMan robot is mounted on a rolling unit. Kinematics of the manipulator are shown in Fig. 2.22. During setup LapMan is registered to the camera trocar using a laser pointer mounted on a part of the robot that is only influenced by the relative positon of the robot to the OR table and the first linear joint. The first linear joint is not used intraoperatively. The three actuated joints are made up of two parallel kinematics and one linear joint at the shaft that attaches to the endoscope. The unconventional design of the LapMan is supposed to improve endoscope motion by locating the camera trocar in the geometric center of the manipulator.

LapMan is controlled by a wireless joystick, named LapStick, which is mounted to a laparoscopic instrument [129].[19] The joystick contains two redundant sets of controls for in/out and left/right motion, the up/down motion is controlled through a distinct 1 DoF flap.

---

[19]Earlier versions of LapMan were controlled by palm interface that was worn under the surgeons glove (cf. [130]).

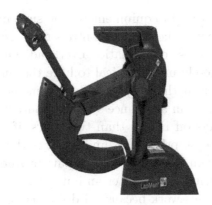

Figure 2.21: The LapMan endoscope manipulator (Source: [128]).

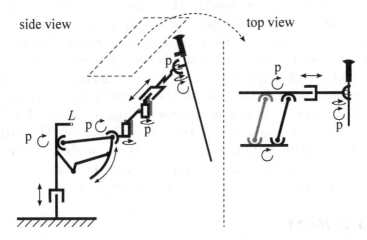

Figure 2.22: Kinematics of the LapMan. The Laser L is used to register robot and trocar. Passive free moving joints are marked with p.

As the title of the paper "How to Maintain the Quality of Laparoscopic Surgery in the Era of Lack of Hands?" by Hourlay [130] already indicates, his focus is on the question how well a human camera assistant can be substituted by a robot. Before going into detail on this question, Hourlay looks at the larger picture in the OR with respect to control of equipment by the surgeon. On one hand, there is an advantage if the surgeon controls more aspects himself, e.g. faster reactions and less coordination overhead. On the other hand, "it would be completely uneconomical to have the surgeon perform all those tasks" given that the surgeon and OR time is a scarce resource. In case of LapMan as an assistance system, Hourlay concludes: First, the investment pays off in less than two years, if the robot is used in 25% of laparoscopic procedures and replaces the human assistant. Second, the stable image contributes to patient safety and increases surgeon's productivity. Third, after an initial learning curve LapMan improves the surgeon's work because of decreased stress level and eye fatigue due to a stable view and autonomy of work.

Tchartchian et al. [128] provides the results of a study in gynecological surgery with 50 patients operated by a single surgeon with robotic assistance and compared to the same number of human-assisted interventions. No statistically significant difference in operative times were found. Further objective results are a lower number of corrections of the endoscope and less time for the manual corrections. In the surgeon's subjective assessment the image stability was also better in the robot-assisted case as well as the satisfaction score. The authors emphasize the improved image stability and the surgeon's autonomy of vision. Finally, concerns are raised about the management of complications in case solo surgery is widely adopted.

2.1.13 SWARM

The SWARM endoscope holder developed in 2005, recently published by Deshparade [131], is a free standing device (Fig. 2.23a) that is controlled by voice or foot pedal. SWARM has four active degrees of freedom in the kinematic configuration shown in Fig. 2.23b. In addition to the usual left/right, up/down, zoom in/out commands diagonal commands have been implemented (for a discussion of this aspect see 2.1.19). The speed of the resulting motion can also be changed by voice. Voice recognition rates of about 95% are reported. Setup times are reported to be as low as 1-2 minutes, although it needs to be covered as it is not sterilizable. In total 784 laparoscopic interventions were performed under SWARM assistance. The author compares SWARM to ViKY and AESOP. In his comparison, SWARM is superior to both other systems in nearly all aspects, such as setup time, task time, voice-control success rate and obstructions.

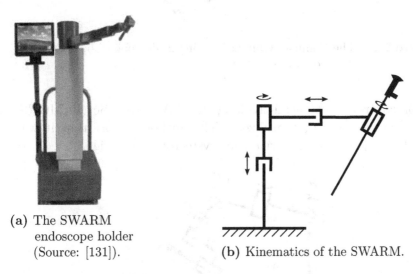

(a) The SWARM endoscope holder (Source: [131]).

(b) Kinematics of the SWARM.

Figure 2.23: The SWARM endoscope holder.

2.1.14 COVER (Compact Oblique-Viewing Endoscope Robot)

The Compact Oblique-Viewing Endoscope Robot (COVER), see Fig. 2.24, aims to exploit oblique-viewing (e.g. 30°) endoscopes to reduce the number of degrees of freedom in endoscope holders [132]. COVER is mechanically positioned over the camera trocar and has three actuated degrees of freedom (Fig. 2.25). Vertical and insertion movements are conventionally implemented by moving the endoscope. However, instead of moving the endoscope horizontally, the authors propose to rotate the oblique-viewing endoscope in order to view different left/right regions.

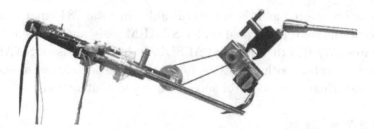

Figure 2.24: The Compact Oblique-Viewing Endoscope Robot (COVER) (Source: [132]).

For control visual head-tracking, the FAce MOUSe (FAMOUS) interface (see p. 89), is utilized. The authors report that it was possible to perform an in vivo cholecystectomy on a pig.

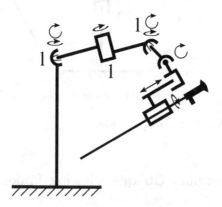

Figure 2.25: Kinematics of the COVER. The first three joints l are mechanically locked during setup time.

2.1.15 SMART (Synthetic Muscle Actuator based Robotic Technology) / P-arm

Taniguchi et al. [133] propose a six DoF endoscope holder based on the kinematics of the Stewart-Gough platform (Fig. 2.27). One version of the system, named SMART (Synthetic Muscle Actuator based

Robotic Technology), uses shape-memory alloy (SMA) as actuators. A later version, named P-arm [134][135][136], uses hydraulic actuators instead (Fig. 2.26). Water is used as fluid in the hydraulic cylinders in order to be biocompatible. The goal for this manipulator is to be very light weight, compact and sterilizable. The authors argue that these attributes, together with accuracy, are best achieved by a parallel structure, such as the chosen Stewart-Gough platform. The endoscope is held in place by a magnetic coupling.

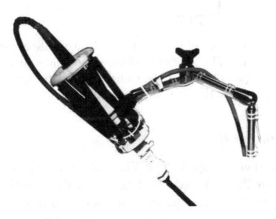

Figure 2.26: The SMART / P-arm endoscope holder (Source: [134]).

In vivo laparoscopic cholecystectomies could be successfully performed on pigs. The endoscope holder was remote controlled by a human camera assistant through a 6 DoF joystick interface, which is also based on a Stewart-Gough platform. The manipulator was found to be about as obstructive as a human camera assistant.

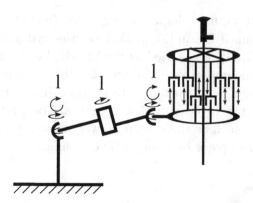

Figure 2.27: Kinematics of the SMART / P-arm (Stewart-Gough platform). The joints l position the actuated part of the endoscope holder over the camera trocar during setup, intraoperatively they are mechanically locked.

2.1.16 Tonatiuh II

The Tonatiuh II endoscope holder (Fig. 2.28a), introduced by Martinez et al. [137] in 2007, Tonatiuh II provides three active degrees of freedom, one freely moving passive joint and two mechanically locked joints for alignment to the camera trocar (Fig. 2.28b). These position the endoscope handle on a sphere around the trocar. The center of the horizontal rotation is aligned with the trocar point during setup of the system. Vertical orientation is achieved by a passive degree of freedom together with translation relative to the trocar point.

The robot is controlled by a gaming joypad. Initial tests in box trainers and animals found that only small forces were exerted at the trocar, even if the endoscope is very close to the abdominal wall. Later on, several clinical tests with different laparoscopic procedures were performed with the Tonatiuh II. Unfortunately, it is unclear whether the surgeon controlled the robot or this was done by an assistant.

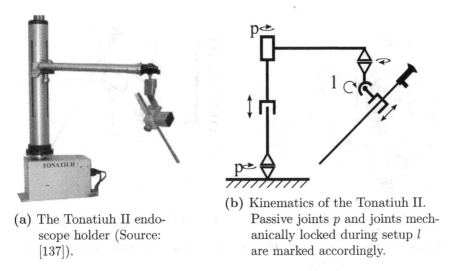

(a) The Tonatiuh II endo-
scope holder (Source:
[137]).

(b) Kinematics of the Tonatiuh II.
Passive joints p and joints mechanically locked during setup l
are marked accordingly.

Figure 2.28: The Tonatiuh II endoscope holder.

2.1.17 PMASS (Postural Mechatronic Assistance Solo Surgery)

The Postural Mechatronic Assistance Solo Surgery (PMASS) [138] is a wearable endoscope holder (Fig. 2.29a) presented in 2009. PMASS is worn by the surgeon like a harness or a simple exoskeleton and provides one actuated degree of freedom and two passive ones (Fig. 2.29b). Weight without endoscope is about 0.5 kg. The actuated joint provides up/down motion of the endoscope and is controlled by a foot switch. Left/right motion and insertion depth is changed by the surgeon rotating his torso respectively moving towards or away from the patient. The two passive joints in conjunction with the trocar point, map these movements to the corresponding endoscope motion.

Initial evaluations were undertaken in veterinary surgery. Reported limitations are restriction to zero-degree optics. Furthermore, one surgeon reported that the equipment and requirement to hold a certain postures results in discomfort in longer procedures. Mishra et al. [139] describe a clinical study undertaken with PMASS. A total of 13 low-

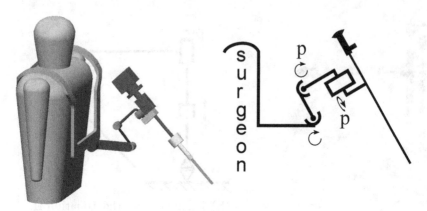

(a) CAD rendering (Source: [138]). **(b)** PMASS kinematics.

Figure 2.29: The wearable Postural Mechatronic Assistance Solo Surgery (PMASS).

risk patients underwent laparoscopic interventions (appendictomies, ovarian cystectomies and sterilizations) performed by three surgeons. Overall the autonomy and ability to control the optics received good and above scores with 4 and higher on a 0 to 5 scale. However, comfort was only judged with 3 to 3.5 points. Shoulder and neck fatigue was criticised as well as a feeling of being tethered to the patient.

2.1.18 FreeHand

The FreeHand camera holder (Fig. 2.30), Prosurgics Ltd., is commercially available since 2009 and the intended successor of the EndoAssist (see p. 35). FreeHand uses head-tracking together with an activation foot switch for control in the same manner as EndoAssist. The surgeon receives visual feedback through a small indicator display showing the recognized motion direction. Motion speed can be adjusted on the robot. The robot is attached to the OR table and positioned by means of a mechanically-locked passive links.[20] In order to register

---

[20]This mechanism is very similar to the one employed by the ViKY endoscope holder (cf. p. 42).

FreeHand's remote center of motion, laser pointer guidance is provided. The actuated part of the kinematics consist of one rotational joint, one C-arch mechanism and a linear joint (Fig. 2.31). In contrast to the ViKY, the motor cables are not free-hanging, but part of the passive linkage.

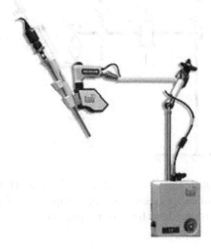

Figure 2.30: The FreeHand endoscope holder (Source: [140]).

Stolzenburg et al. [141] report on a randomized study that compares FreeHand assistance to human assistance in endoscopic extraperitoneal radical prostatectomy (EERPE)[21]. 50 EERPEs were performed by three surgeons, half by robotic assistance and half by human assistance. Human assistance was provided by an inexperienced assistant. No significant difference in operative times were found. The camera robot was faster in horizontal and zooming motions, but slower in vertical ones. Less errors in camera motion were observed and the optics had to be cleaned less often in case of robot assistance. The authors qualify their results with respect to the human assistant by stating that "co-operation between the surgeon and the camera assistant is significantly enhanced when the latter becomes familiar with the

---

[21]Full surgical removal of the prostate gland with access outside the abdominal cavity.

anatomy and the procedure. Thus, the results of the present study may have been different if assistants experienced in camera-holding were compared with the FreeHand".

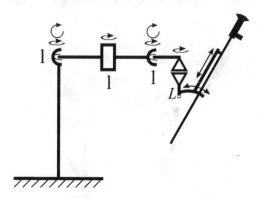

Figure 2.31: Kinematics of the FreeHand. The first three joints l are mechanically locked during setup time. The Laser L is used to register the robot's remote center of motion to the camera trocar.

2.1.19 EVOLAP

Herman et al. [142] developed the EVOLAP endoscope holder (Fig. 2.32) in 2009 with the objectives of high rigidity, low setup time, small footprint at the OR table and flexible placement. The EVOLAP robot is mounted at the OR table. It consists of a parallel mechanism for horizontal and vertical motion located at the edge of the OR table and a linear axis for insertion depth located at the endoscope (Fig. 2.33). The translation of the endoscope handle piece results in a change of orientation due to the combination of the trocar point acting as a pivot point and the two passive joints at the endoscope. A miniature analog joystick that is attached to a laparoscopic instrument is used to control the EVOLAP holder. Fixed and proportional speed control was implemented. Appropriate coordinate system for the joystick control are discussed by the authors and compared those of ViKY,

AESOP and LapMan. An initial in vivo experiment of laparoscopic salpingectomy[22] was successfully completed with EVOLAP assistance.

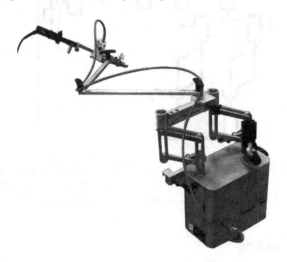

Figure 2.32: The EVOLAP endoscope holder (Source: [143]).

A later study by Herman et al. [143] compares the motion performance of EVOLAP to ViKY and AESOP in box trainer tasks. Also the influence of the mapping from joystick to robot is evaluated. AESOP was found to have the most efficient and intuitive control due to the coordinate frame presented to the user. This was particularly apparent in endoscope positions close to the vertical. Independent of the robot kinematics, a joystick interface that does not only allow three directions of motions, but also diagonal ones was found to improve task performance.

---

[22]The surgical removal of a Fallopian tube.

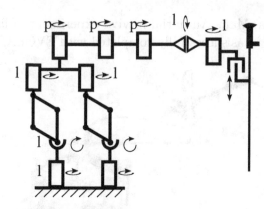

Figure 2.33: Kinematics of the EVOLAP endoscope holder. Only three joints are actuated. Most joints are freely moving passive joints p or mechanically locked during the setup l.

2.1.20 RoboLens

RoboLens is a motorized endoscope holder published by Mirbagheri et al. [144] in 2010. The endoscope positioner is mounted on a cart that is positioned around the OR table. The RoboLens kinematics consist of one linear, two active and one passive rotational joint (Fig. 2.34b). All joints are active, the trocar point is maintained in the robot controller. The authors provide an analysis of the workspaces and manipulability of the RoboLens kinematics. RoboLens can be controlled by a foot pedal and voice commands.

After evaluation of the trajectory following behavior in a lab setting, clinical trials were conducted. RoboLens assisted several surgeons in 30 laparoscopic interventions, most of which were cholecystectomies. The overhead boom allowed to position the bulk part of the endoscope holder away from the surgeon and occupying only the workspace over the camera trocar from above. Although no further details are reported, the authors note that the camera image was stable and no camera cleaning was required. Furthermore, the overall procedure time was lower with robotic camera assistant. Due to issues with the reliability of voice recognition, some surgeons preferred the foot

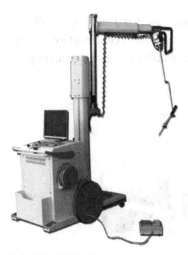

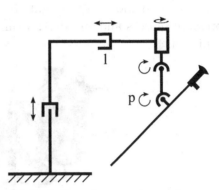

(a) The RoboLens endoscope holder (Source: [144]).

(b) RoboLens kinematics with one passive joint p. The joint marked as l is not in active use intraoperatively.

Figure 2.34: The RoboLens endoscope holder.

pedal interface. At the same time the foot pedal was found to be problematic because of the multiple foot switches that are already used in the OR, e.g. for electrocautery.

2.1.21 Tadano et al.

Tadano et al. [145] introduced a pneumatic laparoscope holder in 2015 (Fig. 2.35). The design is based on a pneumatic surgical manipulator (IBIS IV) developed by the same team [146]. The holder features a remote center of motion, which is implemented by a parallel link mechanism. All four degrees of freedom possible through the camera trocar (cf. Fig. 1.10) are pneumatically actuated. The device is placed over the trocar point and fixed there by mechanical links. The complete structure consists of two rotational joints, one linear and one rotational joint (Fig. 2.36). The second rotational joint is made up of a slider-crank mechanism and actuated by a pneumatic cylinder. Pneumatics are favored for their inherent compliance due to their compressibility and thus safety as well as the possibility to build a compact and more lightweight manipulator. In combination with pressure sensors and encoders, a sufficiently high position accuracy is achieved.

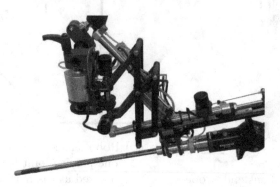

Figure 2.35: The pneumatic endoscope holder by Tadano et al. (Source: [145]).

The endoscope holder is operated through head motions. These are not tracked externally, as with the EndoAssist and FreeHand, but only based gyroscope measurements of two inertial motion sensors (IMU) worn by the surgeon. Robot motion through head movement is only enabled while a foot switch is pressed. Relating to human machine interfaces, the use of a head mounted display (HMD) instead of a conventional monitor is discussed.

Experiments in a box trainer were conducted. The task completion time for simple grasping tasks was similar between human and robot assistance. Finally, the system was also tested in vivo with three gastric resections on pigs. The interventions could be completed with the robotic assistance without lens cleaning.

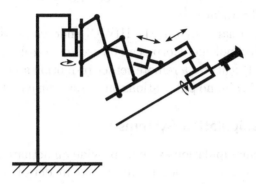

Figure 2.36: Kinematics of the pneumatic endoscope holder. Actuators are two cylinders and two vane motors.

2.1.22 Further systems

The following endoscope holders are summarized in this section because only brief descriptions of the systems are available.

A survey of surgical robotics by Pott et al. [147] from 2005 mentions the Compact Laparoscopic Endoscope Manipulator (CLEM) based on pneumatic muscles and controlled by voice or foot pedal. In addition, the PAROMIS is mentioned, which is based on hexapod kinematics, features force torque sensing and is controlled by speech or touch screen.

In 2009 Kraus et al. [148] describe a system named DeltaScope consisting of Delta kinematics that provide three degrees of translational motion. The trocar serves as fixed point, which alters the translational motion into spherical motions around the trocar point. DeltaScope is operated by joystick. The system was tested in tympanoplasty[23].

The AutoLap image-guided laparoscopic system, Medical Surgery Technologies Ltd., is a compact endoscope holder mounted to the OR table. It provides manual control and instrument tracking based on

---

[23]Surgical reconstruction of the eardrum or small bones.

visual servoing (cf. 2.2.3). Unfortunately, no system description is available in the literature.[24]

Another commercial system is the HIWIN endoscope holder (MTG-H100), HIWIN Technologies Corp., can be used on a trolley or mounted to the OR table. It features a remote center-of-motion and is controlled by a foot pedal. Again, no publications on the system could be found.[25]

2.1.23 Telemanipulation Systems

Although all telemanipulation systems provide an actuated endoscope holder, these systems will not be discussed in detail here for two reasons: First, the scope of this thesis is an assistance system working at the OR table alongside the surgeon. Therefore, surgical telemanipulators in terms of endoscope holding capability do not fall into the intended application domain. Secondly, in a telemanipulation setting the surgeon is already located away from the patient and uses special input devices to control the instruments. Switching between instruments and camera control does not pose as big of an additional obstacle as in conventional MIS. Nevertheless, the knowledge-based endoscope guidance system presented in the following chapters could be directly applied to remote controlled surgical robots.

Rassweiler et al. discuss [149] the cost trade-offs associated with robotic assistance systems for MIS, such as endoscope holders, compared to full telemanipulation setups. Three recent perspectives on remote controlled surgical systems can be found in [150], [151] and [152]. A brief overview of the most well-known telemanipulation systems with a strict focus on their endoscope holding capability and control interface for the endoscope follows.

---

[24]Information about the system is available in a brochure by the manufacturer: http://mst-sys.com/wp-content/uploads/2014/11/AutoLAP_Brochure.pdf.
[25]Information was taken from HIWIN's medical product catalog: http://www.hiwin.tw/download/tech_doc/robot/Medical_Equipment(E).pdf.

da Vinci

The da Vinci [153][33], Intuitive Surgical Inc., is by far the most clinically used surgical robot.[26] The 3D endoscope is mounted to an arm identical in kinematics to the instrument arms, i.e. with a remote center-of-motion and a linear joint for insertion depth. Camera control is performed at the surgeon console by switching control of the input devices from instruments to camera by a foot switch. While the camera is moved the instruments are stationary and vice versa. Nagi et al. developed a low-cost camera arm for the da Vinci Research Kit (dvrk) [155], named CALap.[27]

ZEUS

The ZEUS robotic surgical system [156][157], Computer Motion Inc., was a clinically used system between 1998 and 2003. It consists of three independent manipulators at the patient side. Two of these are remote controlled through hand guided input devices. The third robot is the AESOP (2.1.2) which is controlled by the surgeon via voice using a headset. From a system perspective, the AESOP works as a standalone component. ZEUS was used in the famous first transcontinental robot-assisted laparoscopic cholecystectomy, also known as the "Lindbergh operation" [158].

MiroSurge

The MiroSurge [35] developed by the German Aerospace Center (DLR) is a research system consisting of three independent lightweight robots at the patient side. These robots, named MIRO, share a common ancestry with the KUKA lightweight arms (cf. 4.2.4), however they are much smaller with a reduced payload. Two of the robots are used to position surgical instruments, named MICA, which provide two additional DoFs inside the patient. The third robot positions a conventional endoscope attached to it. The endoscope position and

---

[26]As of September 2015, nearly 3.500 units are installed (Source: [154]).

[27]The da Vinci Research Kit only comprises two manipulator arms by default.

orientation is completely determined by the robot position including rotation along the shaft. Control of the robots is performed through two haptic input devices, Omega.7, Force Dimension. In normal control mode each input device is mapped to one of the instrument robots. To move the endoscope, one input device is used in alternation with instrument control.

RAVEN

The RAVEN surgical robot system [159], Applied Dexterity, is an open research platform consisting of two patient side manipulators with remote center-of-motion kinematics. A particular research focus is long distance telesurgery, e.g. for astronauts on long-term space missions. However, currently only two arms for instrument positioning are part of the RAVEN. Experiments either happen with direct visual observation or use a human camera assistant.

CoBRASurge

The Compact Bevel-geared Robot for Advanced Surgery (CoBRAS-urge) [160][161], is a research system consisting of multiple small robot manipulators. As the name already indicates, CoBRASurge employs a special kinematic based on bevel gears to achieve spherical motion around the trocars in a compact manner. Each manipulator features four degrees of freedom that correspond to those available by the trocar constraint (cf. Fig. 1.10). Instruments and Endoscope are controlled in the same manner by a joystick.

Telelap Alf-X

A recent telesurgical platform is the Telelap Alf-x [162] approved for clinical use in 2012. It has been evaluated in about 150 gynecological interventions. The Telelap Alf-X consists of several large manipulators mounted on wheeled carts that can be individual positioned around the OR table. Long overhead booms allow to move the bulk of the required floorspace for each unit away from the patient, enabling good intraoperative access to the patient. The surgeon controls all robots, at least two for instruments and one for the endoscope, from a surgical console. The instruments are controlled by hand-operated input devices. For control of the 3D endoscope, two interfaces are available: First, an eye-tracking system, which centers the endoscope at the point that the surgeon is looking at on the screen while he presses a button on each input device. Second, zoom and insertion depth change through forward and backward head motion.

2.1.24 Summary

In 1998 Dunlap et al. [163] answer the question whether robotic arms are a cost-effective surgical tool very positively: "The study results indicate the robotic arm not only outperforms human camera holders, but also reduces laparoscopic surgical operating time, resulting in improved efficiency and cost savings to the institution."

Studies that compare human assistance to one of the systems above as well as those that compare two of these have already been described in the previous sections. Arezzo et al. [164] compare the motorized endoscope holders EndoAssist, AESOP and FIPS and the passive mechanical ones, TISKA, Martin arm and Endofreeze in a phantom study.[28] In their results, human assistance always performed best in terms of operative time and all passive systems were superior to the motorized ones.

In a survey on camera and instrument holders from 2004, Jaspers et al. [165] summarize about 70 publications related to passive – PASSIST, Tiska, Martin arm, Unitrack, Ball trocar, Leonard arm – and motorized – AESOP, EndoSista, LapMan, FIPS, Image track camera – endoscope holders. Overall, the literature they surveyed "recognized that using a camera holder in laparoscopic surgery provides an optimal and stable image of the operation field compared with human assistance. The control of the endoscope by the surgeon him/herself is also generally considered to be superior to human assistance. There was no difference in these respects between the

---

[28]The same publication also introduces Endofreeze.

passive and active (robotic) camera holders." At the same time, all interfaces for manual control have clear limitations: There are already multiple foot pedals present in the OR, both hands of the surgeon are already occupied rendering joysticks unergonomic, voice control only allows discrete motions and head control requires artificial head motions. The authors conclude that passive holders appear to work as well or even better than motorized ones and are more cost-efficient.

Feussner et al. state in the context of an overview of technical and digital advancements of surgery from 2014 [166] that motorized endoscope holders clearly failed to gain wide acceptance in the past. Yet, newer systems, such as SOLOASSIST and ViKY, are being reevaluated for their clinical benefits.

In summary, a multitude of endoscope robots have been built in the past 30 years. Many of these were evaluated in animal experiments. Several were evaluated in clinical studies. Nearly ten have been commercialized. Especially for the latter ones, a large number of studies have been published. Table 2.1 summarizes the endoscope holders that were covered in detail above. For the thesis at hand, four aspects are import to note:

- No motorized endoscope holder has reached widespread clinical use.

- Studies clearly show the potential for ergonomic improvements in MIS through usage of endoscope robots.

- A lot of research focused on the evaluation of various kinematics.

- Many interfaces for endoscope control have been researched: foot pedals, joysticks, voice, head, gaze, image pointing and position memory. However, all follow the paradigm of manual control by the surgeon (cf. Fig. 1.8).

Table 2.1: Overview of the motorized endoscope holders described in this section. For joints the following abbreviations are used: Revolute R; Twisting T; Linear L; Universal U; Parallel mechanisms P, e.g. four-bar linkages; and C-arch mechanisms C. Passive free moving joints are marked with a subscript 'p', e.g. R_p. Intraoperative locked joints are marked by a subscript 'l'. $U_l R_l U_l$ often is a standard mechanical instrument holder arm. Note: Telemanipulators and endoscope holders that were not described in detail (2.1.22) are not listed in this table.

Year	System	Robot	Kinematics	Control	References
1993	Endex	Custom	$(5R_p)B_pL$	Foot pedal	[53]
1993	EndoSista		See EndoAssist		[81], [82], [75], [85]
1994	AESOP	Custom	$LRRT_pR_pR$	Backdriving, Foot pedal, Joystick, Position memory, Voice control	[54], [58], [60], [24], [56], [57], [59], [52], [55], [65], [87], [61], [25], [67], [64]
1995	Begin and Hurteau et al.	CRS A460	$(6R)U_p$	Joystick	[68], [69]
1995	LARS / PLRCM	Custom	$LLLPP$	Joystick, Hands-on, Image pointing	[71], [72], [73]
1995	HISAR	Custom	$TRRRTR$	Joystick	[74]

1996	FIPS	Custom	$L_pR_pL_pRCLR$	Finger-ring Joystick, Voice control	[88], [91], [92], [93]
1998	EndoAssist	Custom	LRT	Head-Tracking	[78], [83], [76], [61], [77], [84], [86]
2000	Munoz et al.	Stäubli RX60	$(6R)U_p$	4 DoF Joystick, Voice control	[95], [96]
2001	ERM / Munoz et al.	Custom	$L(2R)(2R_p)$	3D mouse, Voice control	[98], [97], [99], [100], [101]
2002	LER / ViKY	Custom	$U_lR_pU_lRRL$	Backdriving, Foot pedal, Voice control, Position memory	[103], [102], [104], [105], [106], [108], [111], [110], [107], [110], [109]
2003	Naviot	Custom	$P(2R_p)L_p$	Hand control-ler	[112], [113], [114], [116], [115], [117]
2004	LapMan	Custom	$L(2P)LU_p$	Joystick	[127], [130], [129], [128]
2005	SWARM	Custom	$LRLR$	Foot pedal, Voice control	[131]

2006	COVER	Custom	$U_l R_p U_l RLR$	Head-tracking	[132]
2006	SMART / P-arm	Custom	Stewart-Gough	Joystick	[133], [134], [135], [136]
2007	Tonatiuh II	Custom	$R_l LR_l TR_p L$	Joypad	[137]
2008	PMASS	Custom	$R(2R_p)$	Foot pedal and body posture	[138][139]
2009	SOLO-ASSIST	Custom	$T(2R)(2R_p)$	Backdriving, Joystick	[118], [123], [124], [120], [121], [122], [119]
2009	FreeHand	Custom	$U_l R_p U_l RCL$	Head-Tracking	[141]
2009	EVOLAP	Custom	$RPR_p(3R_l) T_p R_p L$	Joystick	[142], [143]
2011	RoboLens	Custom	$LL_l RR_p$	Foot pedal, Voice control	[144]
2014	Tadano et al.	Custom	$RPLR$	Head-Tracking	[145]

2.2 Approaches for Automated Camera Guidance

The previous section comprehensively surveyed motorized endoscope holders. The main focus was on robotic aspects, such as kinematics, the human machine interfaces and suitability for endoscope positioning. Several of these systems will reappear in this section, however, not as motorized endoscope holders under manual control, but as active robots (cf. p. 12). The question is how can positioning of the endoscope – by means of any motorized endoscope holder – be performed autonomously without continuous manual control by the surgeon. As discussed above (cf. 1.1.2), manual control further increases the mental workload of the surgeon. Pandya et al. [167] summarize the problem: "[It] is difficult for the user to obtain optimal camera viewpoints in a dynamic environment or to react effectively to irregular events in the scene due to task overload, latency issues, and complex camera positioning issues. The surgeon has to continually manage the camera position to achieve effective viewpoints through manual control or verbal communication with a second operator."

First related research areas to the automation of endoscope positioning will be briefly discussed, common features and differences will be highlighted. Afterwards a classification of approaches to automated camera guidance is presented. Based on this classification, the approaches known in literature are surveyed.

2.2.1 Related Problems

Active Perception [168] explores strategies for active acquisition of perceptional information. Instead of relying on a sensory system with fixed properties, expertise about sensors, reproduction properties and the information gathering task are employed to create a system that actively adapts to external circumstances. Which information is gathered does not simply depend on contingencies about the external makeup of the environment, but is gathered purposefully with respect to the data acquisition task.

For visual perception, Active Vision [169] looks at an observer that is able to change geometric parameters of the scenery. In relation to robotics, this usually means that the visual sensor can change position within the environment or manipulate the environment by rearranging objects. Many visual ambiguities about object properties can be easily resolved, if sensory information from multiple direction can be captured. A simple perspective example is shown in Fig. 2.37: Resolving the spatial ambiguities without getting different perspectives must rely on very minute details or can be impossible altogether. If the scene can be explored, i.e. viewed from different points, the actual spatial relations can be recognized.

The problem of Next Best View [170] is a sequence of view points to achieve a given vision task. For example, it is not possible to obtain a complete spatial model of most scenes from a single view point due to occlusions. "Next" is part of the problem name because the time component of the problem becomes important when executed on physical systems that have to move through space. Not only the more apparent minimization of total path length is a reason, but also that some view sequences could not be possible or dangerous.

Active Perception, Active Vision and Next Best View are insofar quite different from automated camera guidance that problems are often posed as (a series of) offline problems[29]. Camera guidance is an assistance function performed in real-time alongside the actions of the surgeon. Thus, the target objective of the perception task change together with the surgical task. To some extent the same holds true for the environment, which is constantly changing over the course of the intervention. This is especially true with respect to the surgical instruments, which are the most salient feature of task and environment.

Another related problem is control of virtual cameras in computer graphics, e.g. computer games. However, there are many differences between positioning a virtual camera and a real (endoscope) camera. First of all, in the virtual environment the camera placement algorithm has access to the ground truth about the position of all scene objects. Secondly, the virtual camera is not constrained by physical limitations, for example in terms of (re)positioning velocity. Thirdly, it is assumed that the optimal camera position is already

---

[29]The term 'offline problem' is derived from the distinction between offline and online algorithms. Offline algorithms have access to the full problem statement from the beginning, e.g. the input data. Online algorithms on the other hand receive the input piecewise while doing computation on the already received data.

specified by a set of constraints or a known cost function. Therefore, none of the approaches can be directly applied to real-world endoscope positioning. The overview paper by Christie et al. [171] provides many more details on this subject.

As shown in the survey by Kober et al. [172] the field of reinforcement learning is widely applied to learning tasks in the domain of robotics. In reinforcement learning the system explores different strategies and receives rewards depending on its task success. However, the paradigm seems unsuitable to train an endoscope robot for the following reasons: First, the reward function must be engineered before the system can start to learn. Yet, this either presupposes already having a model of good endoscope positions, which is actually part of the learning task, or requires the use of very coarse reward functions. In the latter case, too many interventions would be required until the system behavior converges. In general, even if safety issues would be solved, there are significant practical obstacles with respect to the number of interventions required for training. Most case studies on reinforcement learning in robotics require on the order of 100 episodes to learn short dynamic tasks. This poses a big obstacle to apply the methods in the context of surgical robotics research, where recording and annotation of 10 interventions is already a major effort. In contrast, as shown in chapter 7, already five recorded interventions can be enough to train the system presented in this thesis for a 25 minute intervention.

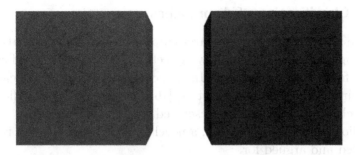

(a) From this perspective the cube on the left appears to have the same size as the cube on the right. Both seem to be next to each other and have the same distance from the virtual camera.

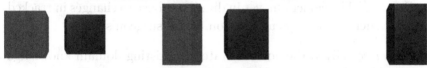

(b) From left to right the observer approaches the two blocks straight ahead. It soon becomes obvious that the blocks are neither next to each other nor have the same size.

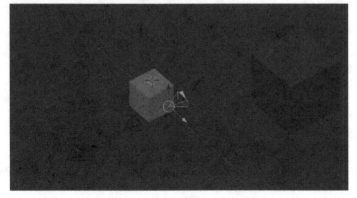

(c) Orthographic view of the actual scene: The left block is half the size and far in front of the right block. The four positions of the virtual camera for the images above are also indicated.

Figure 2.37: Illustration how active vision can easily resolve scene ambiguities that cannot be easily resolved from a single perspective.

2.2.2 Classification of Approaches

For the survey of current research approaches to the automation of endoscope guidance in the following section, a systematic classification is put forth in this section. In a recent survey paper on camera viewpoint automation Pandya et al. [167] propose such a classification. Their classification will be described next. However, due to the limitations of this classification, a novel extended classification is then proposed and argued for.

The top-level partition proposed by Pandya et al. is between reactive, proactive and combined control strategies (cf. Fig. 2.38):

- *Reactive*: The camera moves in direct response to changes in tracked data, such as instrument position or the surgeon's gaze.

- *Proactive*: Given the current state, preexisting domain knowledge is employed to predict the best camera position.

- *Combined*: Control has aspects of reactive and proactive control.

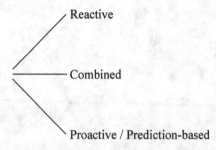

Figure 2.38: Classification of viewpoint automation proposed by Pandya et al.

The classification for automation of camera positioning proposed here is two-dimensional and structured as follows (cf. Fig. 2.39): First dimension (A):

- *Direct*: A simple algorithmic mapping between current features and camera motion. Features can be simple, e.g. position of instrument tip, or complex, e.g. surgical gestures[30].

  - *General-purpose*: The algorithmic mapping can be directly applied to other camera positioning problems.

  - *Domain-specific*: The algorithmic mapping was specifically designed for the task domain and does not easily translate to other tasks.

- *Model-based*: Camera motion depends on a model that is part of the algorithms input data, i.e. given the same scene information, but with a different model will significantly alter the camera motion.[31]

  - *Reactive*: The resulting motion depends only on the current point in time.

  - *Planned*: The resulting motion depends on a time interval. This can include a memory of past states or planning ahead by means of a simulation model.

Second dimension (B):

- *Constant*: The system always uses the same mapping between input and camera motion.

- *Context-aware*: The system changes the mapping depending on a high-level property such as intervention type or surgical task.

Thus an approach must be assigned one class from each dimension A and B, e.g. an approach can be "constant, direct general-purpose" or "context-aware, model-based planned".

---

[30]A surgical gesture, or surgeme, is located between the task level, e.g. suturing, and motion primitives (cf. [173]).

[31]To explicitly deny the loop hole of simply loading a 'direct' program as data (into an interpreter) and referring to this as 'model-based', the following restriction must hold: The loaded model must not be Turing complete.

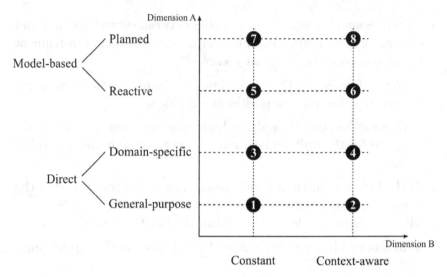

Figure 2.39: Proposed two-dimensional classification of camera automation.

2.2.3 Survey of Approaches

Employing the classification proposed in the previous section, existing approaches to camera automation will be summarized and classified in this section.[32] In order to keep the survey focused and at a reasonable length, papers that deal with the automation of other laparoscopic tasks, e.g. suturing, are excluded, even though some apply similar methods. Publications are sorted into the categories and described chronologically within each category.

Direct General-purpose (1,2)

Visual Servoing Visual Servoing is a particularly prominent direct general-purpose approach. Therefore, this approach will first be described in general terms without reference to specific publications. Afterwards, all publications that employ visual servoing can

---

[32]The numbers of the following subsections correspond to those in Fig. 2.39.

be described more concisely with reference to this general description. Publications that only treat instrument detection and tracking, but do not apply it for automated endoscope positioning are briefly discussed in 5.2.1.

Visual Servoing refers to the process of tracking a feature in an image stream, comparing the feature's current position to a desired position and moving an actuator in order to reduce the distance between current and desired feature position. Fig. 2.40 illustrates this principle. In order to reduce the alignment error in each timestep[33], the kinematical relation between change of robot position and the camera's field of view must be known. If robot dynamics can be ignored in the outer control loops – which is assumed here given the low accelerations and velocities required for endoscope motion, often a velocity-based control approach is employed. Given a transformation between robot and camera coordinates, the time derivatives of the image coordinates can be written as a Jacobian matrix J. The (pseudo-)inverse of the Jacobian J^{-1} can then be used to compute the robot motion for the next time step δq from the alignment error in the image δp.

For more details, Azizian et al. [174][175] provide an extensive survey on visual servoing in medical robotics. An older but complementary article is available by Groeger et al. [176].

Approaches The pioneering work in 1994 by Lee and Uecker et al. [177][178][179] implemented markerless visual servoing on the AESOP (cf. 2.1.2). The term 'markerless' refers here to the use of standard laparoscopic instruments that were not modified in any manner, e.g. through the addition of colored rings at their distal end.[34] Further information on the instrument detection and tracking can be found in section 5.2.1. Given the position of the instrument

---

[33]Cameras typically provide 30 images per second, assuming features can be detected at this frame rate of 30 Hz, the gap to the much higher robot control rates (100 - 1000 Hz) must be bridged by interpolation. The arising problems of cascade control will not be addressed here.

[34]A corresponding distinction is between natural and artificial landmarks.

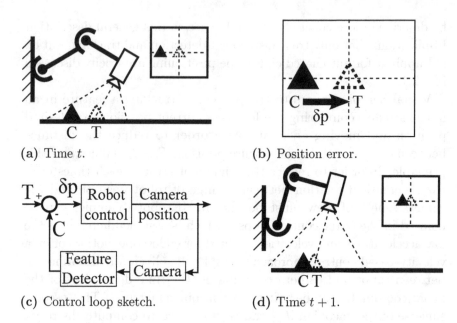

(a) Time t.   (b) Position error.

(c) Control loop sketch.   (d) Time $t + 1$.

Figure 2.40: A simple example of Visual Servoing. The robot position is changed in each timestep in order to make the current feature position C coincidence with the target feature position T.

tip, the authors propose a velocity controller based on the inverse Jacobian that keeps an instrument tip in the center of the image. Only left/right and up/down motion was implemented, insertion depth is manually controlled by the surgeon. The approach is classified as general-purpose because the model is directly applicable to visual servoing tasks outside surgery. The system is not context-aware.

A US patent by Kudo et al. [180] from 1998 describes an endoscope positioning system that tracks instruments by means of color markers or by electromagnetic three-dimensional position sensors. Servoing of orientation and zoom is performed. Furthermore, the system comprises different manual control interfaces such as a joystick, head-tracking and position memory.

Zhang et al. [181] present monochrome markers for instrument tracking in 2002, realized as strips along the endoscope shaft. They elaborate on the peculiarities of camera calibration for endoscopes because the marker shape together with an intrinsically well calibrated endoscope can provide depth information from monocular images. Experiments showed that the markers were robust to specular reflections and could be tracked well. Unfortunately, no experimental results for the visual servoing performance are provided.

The master thesis of Sivadasan [182] from 2006 compares the mental workload and task completion time between eye gaze and joystick control in a simple lab setup. The subjective workload according to the NASA Task Load Index (TLX) questionnaire for a simple camera aiming task was lower for gaze control. Task performance was very similar to joystick control.

Bourger et al. [183] apply the model-free efficient second-order minimization (ESM[35]) tracking algorithm based on histogram matching. The method is insofar MIS specific as the trocar constraint (Fig. 1.10) is incorporated into the servoing control. However, all other aspects can be directly applied to other visual servoing tasks. In particular, the histogram-based tracking is directly applicable for tracking outside of the surgical context. Results with AESOP (cf. 2.1.2) in a box trainer showed relatively slow convergence attributed to a significant amount of noise in the histogram matching, non-linearities in camera positioning and the high latency of the AESOP controller.

Polski et al. [185] describe servoing of the SOLOASSIST (cf. 2.1.11) by means of electromagnetic trackers in 2009. Markers are attached to the endoscope camera and the instrument. The servoing task evaluated in a test box was to keep a fixed distance between the endoscope tip and the instrument tip. Positioning accuracy was between 10 mm and 30 mm depending on size of the test target. Motion hysteresis

---

[35]Mali [184] formulates visual servoing as minimization problem and employs results of the latter to the former. In analogy to the use of a first-order Tayler series approximation in the Gauss-Newton method (GNM) for minimization, a second-order Taylor series is used for ESM.

(Fig. 2.41) was used to keep the endoscope position stable for small instrument motions.

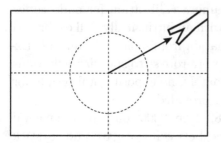

(a) Instrument distance above hysteresis threshold (dashed circle): Camera moves.

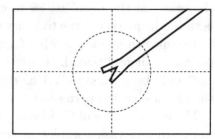

(b) Camera has centered on instrument tip – assuming this being the optimal position.

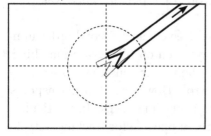

(c) Instrument moves, but new distance below hysteresis threshold.

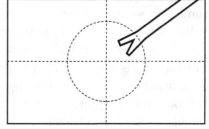

(d) Camera remains still until instrument leaves hysteresis region.

Figure 2.41: Illustration of motion hysteresis to stabilize camera position.

In 2010 Osa et al. [186] implement visual servoing of the endoscope on a telemanipulation system, named Endo[PA]R[36]. Special attention is given to a modified interaction matrix that takes the coupling between linear and angular velocities into account, which is due to the trocar constraint (Fig. 1.10). Apart from this, standard visual

---

[36]The Endoscopic Partlally-Autonomous Robot (Endo[PA]R) system [187] consists of four ceiling mounted Mitsubishi MELFA 6SL robots equipped with force-torque sensors.

servoing with color markers on the instruments is used for automatic camera control.

Noonan et al. [188] describe gaze contingent control for an endoscope with additional degrees of freedom at the endoscope tip in 2010. Since the flexible instruments are outside the scope of this survey, only the control aspects that generalize to the control of a conventional rigid endoscope will be explained. A stand-alone eye tracker, Tobii x50, records the 2D fixation points on a monitor at 50 Hz. The surgeon must keep his head in a volume of $30 \times 16 \times 20$ cm in front of the screen. To control the endoscope motion, the screen is split into five regions: a central area and the four corner quadrants. After selecting a GUI button by fixation, the endoscope rotates towards the four image corners until the central area is fixated again. Motion speed is selected by the distance from the screen center. To rotate along the endoscope shaft the surgeon has to first fixate on a GUI button and afterwards move the endoscope by fixating on the left or right part of the screen. Evaluation was performed by a pointing task in a box trainer, but not compared to other control modalities.

King et al. [189] describe automatic instrument tracking in a lab test setup consisting of a box trainer and a pan-tilt-zoom webcam in 2013. Color markers are attached to the instrument tips. Based on the instrument tip position, the following rules have been implemented: If two instruments are visible, the camera is centered between their tips. Motion hysteresis is used to reduce the amount of camera motion as long as the tips are sufficiently close to the image center. If both instruments are close to the image center, the camera zooms in and out if they are too close to opposing image edges. No motion is performed if no or only one instrument is visible.

Lie and Zhang et al. [190][191] present gaze control of the CoBRAS-urge endoscope holder (cf. 2.1.23) in 2013. A stand-alone eye tracking system, S2 Eye Tracker, is used to acquire the gaze data at 60 Hz in a working volume of $25 \times 11 \times 30$ cm. After low-pass filtering of the raw gaze data, fixations lasting for 2 seconds are detected. If the surgeon confirms the intent[37] to move the endoscope by a foot clutch the fixation point is used to reposition the endoscope accordingly. The authors report that a simple pointing task in a box trainer could be performed by multiple users.

Building on their earlier work (cf. p. 2.2.3), in 2015, Li et al. [193] present gaze control that distinguishes natural eye movement from control intended eye movement based on fuzzy logic. The automatic classification between gaze for control and gaze for observation was evaluated by visual exploration tasks in a box trainer. Compared with the earlier approach based on pure dwell time, the fuzzy interface had a better average response time (1.4 to 2.1 seconds), but with a higher variation. In a subjective assessment conducted through a usability questionnaire, the fuzzy interface scored better (100 to 88.5 points on a scale from 0 to 130), yet, the dwell time interface was found slightly superior for repetitive tasks.

Direct Domain-specific (3,4)

In 1997 Wei et al. [194][195] published a visual servoing approach based on color markers attached to the instruments in combination with a stereo laparoscope.[38] The AESOP 1000 (cf. 2.1.2) robot was used for endoscope positioning. All three degrees of freedom are determined by the visual servoing control. The insertion depth, i.e. the distance to the instrument tips, was determined by means of stereo disparity of the detected color markers. Motion gain for small image displacements was set to a low value in order to have a stable static image position. Furthermore, the detected instrument positions were low-pass filtered in the temporal and spatial domain. So far the algorithm is general-purpose, however, additional domain-specific rules that address characteristics of MIS are employed, too: The robot will not immediately change the endoscope position, when a

---

[37]The problem with gaze control is that control is always 'on' because the surgeon does not only look at the screen in order to interact with it, but also to just see its content (cf. [192]).

[38]A patent for the procedure was filed in 1996 [196].

new instrument enters the field of view. Normal instrument motion is distinguished from motions such as retraction of the instrument by manual thresholds. In the latter case, the robot will not follow the instrument. However, the control rules are not context-aware and constant throughout the intervention. An evaluation in pigs showed that the system followed the instruments well, even if they were partially occluded, stained or vision was deteriorated by smoke caused by electrocautery[39]. The authors argue that adding color-marks to laparoscopic instruments would have negligible cost and not impact their surgical properties. In 1999 Omote et al. [197] report the application of the system, named Self-Guided Robotic Camera Control for Laparoscopic (SGRCCS), in 20 laparoscopic cholecystectomies and compared these to 58 human-assisted ones. Setup time of the system was 21 minutes on average, 83% of the procedures could be completed with SGRCCS assistance. Average operative times with the robot were 54 minutes and 60 minutes without robot assistance. Furthermore, a reduced number of corrective camera movements and lens cleanings are reported for robot assistance. The subjective assessment in comparison to human assistance favored the robot in 12 cases, found it to be equally good in three cases and worse in two.

The line of research started in 2001 by Nishikawa et al. [198] looks into head control of endoscopes by means of visual face tracking. After the initial publication the system was named FAce MOUSe, or FAMOUS. The first method described is based on iris detection from a grayscale image provided by a camera mounted to the monitor that displays the endoscopic video. A second method recognizes a black marker tape that is attached to the surgical cap. The following interaction method assumes that the surgeon remains in a constant distance to the screen and faces it in parallel. Pan and zoom motions are initiated by different face gestures. If the surgeon tilts his head first left then right the pan mode is initiated, if he performs these motions the other way round zoom mode is toggled. In each mode

---

[39]Cauterization, the selective burning of tissue, by means of electrically generated heat.

left/right and up/down rotation of the surgeon's head determines the relative motion speed of the endoscope. A finalizing head gesture stops endoscope control. An in vivo experiment, laparoscopic cholecystectomy on a pig, could be performed without a human assistant and no lens cleaning was required. During the 44 minute intervention, 97 face motions had to be performed by the surgeon. In 2002 the system was compared to a voice control interface [199] using the Virtual Laparoscopic Interface (VLI), Immersion Corporation, which simulates simple laparoscopic manipulations and is controlled by two mechanically tracked laparoscopic instruments and a foot pedal. Three tasks used in the evaluation were derived from actual surgical actions performed during cholecystectomy, but much simplified: retrieval of gallbladder, dissection and ligation of cystic duct and vessels, dissection of gallblader from liver. Suitability of the endoscope view was scored by rate of compliance to the rule that the target must be within a fixed distance to the endoscope and sufficiently close to the center of the image. No significant difference in task completion time were found. The amount of time spend for camera manipulation and endoscope path distance were smaller with face control. On the other side, instrument paths were longer and task errors were more frequent with face control. In an extended article from 2003 [200], the analogy between face control and mouse control, giving FAce MOUSe its name, is expounded. Also further details on the custom endoscope holder are provided, which employs kinematics that are similar to the LARS robot (cf. 2.1.4). In addition, more in vitro experiments are described. The system was also compared to instrument tracking in a two box trainer interventions with pig organs [201]. Qualitatively, instrument tracking was found to be problematic for very fine manipulations with high zoom.

Voros et al. [202][203] exploit the special geometric layout of MIS in the abdomen (cf. Fig. 1.2) in 2006. It is known that both camera and instruments enter the abdominal cavity through the trocar points located on the surface defined by the inflated abdominal wall. These points can be measured by means of a calibrated endoscope robot. The diameter of the laparoscopic instrument's shaft is also known.

Calibration includes intrinsic camera calibration and extrinsic, hand-eye, camera to robot calibration. The trocar points are viewed from two different positions by the manually controlled endoscope robot. Because the transformation between the recording positions is known, conventional stereo vision algorithms can be used to compute the 3D location from the 2D images. This information is projected on to the image plane and simplifies finding the instrument axis and instrument tip in the image. For experimental purposes the ViKY endoscope holder is used. Instrument detection results from a cadaver experiment show a detection error of less than 11 pixels for a 200×100 pixel image resolution in 87% of the images. However, systematic wrong detections are reported, too. No visual servoing results are provided.

The master thesis by Munduri [204] from 2010 implements two automatic camera modes on the ZEUS telemanipulator (cf. 2.1.23). Based on the known transformation between the three robotic arms deployed in the ZEUS system together with a registration of the trocar points, the instrument position is known from the forward kinematics. Given the endoscope and instrument position, a zoom mode and a following mode are implemented. The zoom mode calculates the angle between camera center and the instrument in order to keep it visible ($< 35°$) and not too close ($> 15°$). In following mode, the algorithm tries to keep the endoscope centered on the instrument. Motion speed is low in order to avoid too much motion. Switching between static, zoom and following mode is performed manually.

Song et al. [205] base their approach on tracking of color markers at the instrument tip. The image distance between instruments is used to determine the zoom ratio. Yet, the authors note that since this measure is based on the image distance only, the distance for instruments with different depths can be easily misjudged. As a workaround a second color marker was attached to the instrument that must be within the field of view, thus keeping a minimum distance between endoscope and instruments. Experiments were performed with a Webcam on a pan-tilt unit. Motion hysteresis is used for tracking stabilization.

Yu et al. [206] describe automatic positioning of the endoscope in the Laparoscopic Minimally Invasive Surgical Robotic System (LMISRS) telemanipulation system in 2013. Their algorithm is based on the known position of the endoscope and telemanipulated instruments. Given an initial view angle of the instruments, the authors elaborate on the kinematic transform required to keep the endoscope in the same view angle while the instruments move. No experimental results for the servoing scheme are provided.

In 2013 Fujii et al. [207] present gaze control of an endoscope by means of explicit gaze gestures. The authors favor gaze gestures because of the inherent intentional ambiguity provided by eye motion. Other works have to use an additional input channel, such as a foot pedal, for disambiguation in gaze control. Recognition of gestures is achieved by modeling each one as a Hidden Markov Model (HMM). The forward-back algorithm is used to assign a probability to each HMM for a given observation. The most likely gesture is then selected. Two gestures for zoom and pan were trained and evaluated. The system is evaluated in a box trainer with a KUKA LWR IV (cf. 4.2.4) that positions the endoscope. Cartesian impedance control is employed to provide force-torque constrained positioning. The trocar constraint is obeyed by specifying sufficient intermediate poses that are followed in a point-to-point (PTP) manner by the controller. Once an eye gesture is recognized, a GUI is overlaid on the laparoscopic image. The actual zoom or pan is then determined through the eye fixture on the screen. Activation of zoom and pan mode by gaze gestures was compared to activation by foot pedals. Gaze control was used in both cases. Eleven surgical residents took part in the box trainer experiments. The first task consisted of navigating the endoscope on a numbered grid. The second task was to remove a set of 'lesions' in an upper gastrointestinal phantom, which required bimanual manipulation. As control group to the gaze gesture and the foot pedal activated gaze control, conventional human assistance was evaluated. Assessment comprised task time and camera path length as well as the NASA TLX questionnaire on mental task load. Robot assistance in both modes was found to result in significantly shorter camera paths compared to human assistance. Task completion time did not differ between all three modes. Although the median score for mental load in case of foot pedal activation was lower, the difference was not significant. The score for robot and human assistance did not differ significantly either.

In their paper from 2014, Zhao et al. [208] combine the instrument markers by Zhang et al. (cf. p. 85) with the geometrical method by Voros et al. (cf. p. 90) for visual servoing with the ViKY endoscope holder (cf. 2.1.9). Given the acquired trocar points in 3D relative to the instrument trocar and an intrinsically calibrated endoscope, the 2D marker position in the image can be triangulated to 3D positions. The reconstructed positions are smoothed by a Kalman filter for tracking. Visual servoing of all three actuated degrees of freedom provided by the ViKY is performed. No experimental results beyond the tracking accuracy are provided.

Model-based Reactive (5,6)

In 1996 Casals et al. [209] describe situation-dependent camera control by means of visual servoing using tracked instruments that are marked with two straight lines along the tool axis. The tool diameter in the endoscopic image is used to approximate the distance between endoscope and tool tip. Three surgical situations are distinguished to have the same camera control rules: two moving surgical instrument in the scene; one moving and one relatively steady auxiliary instrument in the scene; only a single instrument visible in the scene. In case of two active instruments, the endoscope is positioned in the middle of the line connecting the two instrument tips. In case of one dominant instrument, the endoscope is also positioned on the line connection both instrument tips, however, not in the middle but closer to the dominant one. Finally, in case of a single instrument in the scene, the camera centers on the predicted next position of the instrument tip. Zoom is controlled to keep the instrument(s) in the field of view, but since the optimal zoom depends on the surgeon's preferences, control is done relative to an initial parameter set by the surgeon. Filtering is applied in order to smooth the endoscope motion. The implemented filter mixes motion hysteresis (cf. Fig 2.41) with a gain proportional to the position error. In case of large deviations that risk the tool disappearing from the camera view, direct tracking is used. Thus the approach can be characterized as context-aware and model-based reactive (see number 6 in Fig. 2.39). The system was evaluated in the operating room on a commercial robot [210], unfortunately, no detailed results are reported.

Nishikawa et al. [211] describe a system based on preoperative workspace planning combined with intraoperative instrument servoing in 2006. Preoperatively, the surgeon manually defines workspaces in the abdominal cavity which determine the desired zoom ratio. Intraoperatively, when an instrument enters the predefined workspaces the endoscope is centered on the instrument tip with the respective zoom ratio. Between multiple workspaces the zoom ratio is linearly interpolated. Instruments are externally tracked by a Polaris system, NDI. Qualitative results, from a laparoscopic cholecystectomy in a box trainer with pig organs, showed that the adaptive change of the zoom ratio was well received. However, the implementation, due to a multitude of defined workspaces within the working area of the instrument, changed the zoom ratio too frequently. Since the manual definition of workspaces takes surgical phases into account, this approach can be considered context-aware.

In 2008 Nishikawa et al. [212] present a system that acquires the optimal zoom ratio by observing previous interventions. By means of externally tracked instruments, Polaris, NDI, the distance and angle between the laparoscope and instruments were recorded in a box trainer. The authors look at the correlation between angle and distance and use this relation as control law in visual servoing. The angle-distance control law was compared to a fixed-distance control law in a box trainer for cholecystectomy on pig organs.

Rivas-Blanco et al. [213] present automated camera positioning based on a cognitive architecture in 2014. The lab setup consists of a Barret WAM arm with 7 DoFs, both tracked by an external marker-based tracking system, Polaris, NDI, together with a box as abdomen phantom. Instead of a laparoscope, the camera is held on the inside of the abdominal wall by a magnet at the robot end effector. The robot translates the camera along the abdominal wall instead of changing its orientation as for a conventional endoscope. However, the details of this hardware setup are disregarded in the following explanation of the control system. A cognitive architecture comprised of short-term and long-term memory is proposed by the authors. The long-term memory consists of a semantic memory that stores information about interventions and surgical facts, a procedural memory that stores learned behaviors and an episodic memory that stores experiences of the user. In the short-term memory the surgical state is estimated (cf. 5.2.2) and the focus of attention (FOA) is estimated that in turn triggers a motion behavior of the camera. The human-machine interface (HMI) enables the surgeon to adapt the manually the camera view. For each surgical gesture known to the system a trained Hidden Markov Model (HMM) is used for recognition. The position of an object in the camera image together with the zoom factor, referred to as FOA, is specified for each state of a surgical task. This mapping is individualized for each surgeon over time: Every time the surgeon gives a voice command to manually change the camera position, the modified relation is associated with the current surgical task. The system was evaluated by five non-experts performing a suturing task in the lab setting described above. After three trials with manual control of the camera position by voice, the same task was again performed three times with automated camera positioning. While a large reduction in the number of voice commands is reported, the overall task time was not significantly reduced.[40] The camera motion employs a model of the intervention, is context-aware of the surgical task and uses reactive visual servoing.

In 2014 Agustinos et al. [214] continue the approach by Voros et al. (cf. p. 90), making it context-aware and implementing it on the ViKY endoscope holder (cf. 2.1.9). Based the recognition

---

[40]Since the trials were not performed in random order, the learning which is to be expected in novices was not accounted for.

of the current surgical step in a workflow model, different tracking modes are activated:[41] With a single single instrument in the scene its tip is tracked with or without motion hysteresis (cf. Fig. 2.41). In case of several instruments present, either one of these is tracked, which assumes they can be reliably distinguished without markers, or the intersection point of their shaft axis is used as tracking target. Experiments were performed in a box trainer that showed that visual tracking converges, but without motion filtering the camera image can become unstable due to tracking noise. The latter is especially a problem when the intersection between two instrument is tracked due to the projective error enlargement.

Model-based Planned (7,8)

Wang et al. [215][216] present a system in 1996 that incorporates high-level models, planned scope motions and reactive motions based on image processing. The system comprises several conceptual layers (from top to bottom): supervising & planning, guidance & control, integration & coordination and sensing & modeling. The authors characterize the system as "choreographed" because sequences of actions can be executed semi-automatically. Initial trocar insertion is given as an example. The surgeons initiates the sequence by voice command, image analysis and object recognition are then used to ground each step. First, the endoscope is positioned towards the abdominal wall, visual analysis focuses on bulging parts in the image and recognizes when the trocar tip penetrates the abdominal wall. Different voice commands initiate manual motion of the endoscope or visual servoing to an instrument tip (cf. Lee and Uecker et al. on p. 83). The high-level plans allow to specify different reactive behaviors of the lower levels, thus the system is context-aware.

Starting in 2004, Ko and Kwon et al. [217][218][219] describe interaction with the endoscope robot[42] based on a surgery task model.

---

[41] The authors refer to known approaches for phase identification in the literature, autonomous mode switching is not actually implemented.

[42] The KaLAR robot featuring a custom bendable endoscope is used.

The robot should not only react to direct commands, but autonomously respond to the surgeon's actions and the current task. Although the main purpose of a task model is better human-robot interaction (HRI), it also facilitates environment perception. The surgery task model consists of states (surgical stages), transitions triggered by environment information and an action strategy associated with each state. Transitions can be probabilistic, accounting for variance in procedures. An example model of laparoscopic cholecystectomy is provided by the authors. For camera assistance, each tuple of state and instrument is manually assigned with the preferred camera mode, which can be either static, voice commands or visual servoing of an instrument. Instruments are augmented by different color markers that are used for tracking of the instrument and identification of its type. A further mode that the authors plan to implement is automatic centering on an anatomical region. The system was in vivo evaluated by three cholecystectomies in small pigs. Average operating time was 26.7 minutes, which is put in relation to the surgeon's average times in human cholecystectomies of 23.3 minutes. The automatic selection of the preferred camera mode was found to reduce the number of voice commands from 71 to 50.

The autonomous endoscope guidance described by Weede et al. [220][221] in 2011 builds on a knowledge base of recorded interventions from one intervention type. All trajectories undergo a clustering algorithm that distributes a predefined number of cluster centers over the data points that minimize the distance between points to their clusters. Once the clusters have been positioned and data points assigned to them, the covariance of each cluster is determined. In the next step, each trajectory is traversed and the transition between different clusters are recorded. The resulting transition probabilities between clusters in turn are used to define a second-order Markov chain that encodes a probabilistic trajectory through the combined interventions. In order to capture the important relation between the two instruments, the points corresponding to each instrument tip are represented as a combined six dimensional vector. Intraoperatively the current position of the instruments is assigned to a cluster by means of a maximum likelihood classifier. The Markov chain is then used to predict the most likely next cluster to which the instruments will move. Based on a set of manually defined rules for an optimal endoscopic field of view, the camera is moved, if the prediction finds one instrument outside this view. To increase motion smoothness, the resulting camera positions are spatially low-pass filtered. The authors evaluated the prediction performance in a box trainer where different landmarks hand to be touched in three defined sequences with laparoscopic instruments. On average the prediction was accurate with between 89.1% to 92.3% depending on the number of clusters specified. Compared to a purely reactive camera positioning, 29% less camera motions were required. The approach is model-based planned and constant as the relation between camera position and instruments is manually specified and independent of the current surgical task.

In an abstract from 2013 Bauer et al. [222] describe the "soloassist-cognitive" project. The project's aim is to combine eye tracking control and visually tracked instruments for partially autonomous camera positioning based on a model of the surgical workflow. Unfortunately, no further details on the project are currently available. Two of the Fundamentals of Laparoscopic Surgery (FLS) manual skill tests[43], namely peg transfer and precision cutting, were modified to require camera repositioning. The pegs were placed further apart and the circle was enlarged that had to be cut. No quantitative results are provided, but the authors report the automatic camera positioning to be well suited for the tasks. Furthermore, the authors recognize that the "presented camera system currently has a very basic movement scheme that essentially keeps both instruments in the camera's view at all times. This corresponds to the simplest instruction that could be given to a novice camera holder. Such a movement scheme may be adequate in some situations, but it is not ideal or sufficient for many tasks."

---

[43]These are comprised of peg transfer, pattern cut, ligating loop, extracorporeal suture and intracorporeal suture [11].

Summary

Table 2.2 summarizes all approaches detailed above. The majority of approaches either focuses on improving manual control modalities or looks into visual servoing strategies. Several approaches include context-awareness based on a model of the surgical workflow that modifies the underlying control strategies, e.g. a different zoom level is assigned to each surgical step. There is a clear correlation between model-based approaches and context-awareness. In terms of Fig. 2.39, the bottom-left (1,3) and the top-right (6,8) are dominant. Authors that recognize a need for endoscope control that is not derived from hand coded direct algorithms, but employs a model of the surgical task, also recognize the requirement for adaptation to different surgical tasks. In general, there is a lack of meaningful evaluation and comparison of different methods. Lacking a benchmark or at least a clear agreement on a protocol to evaluate these approaches, progress in the field of automated camera positioning or viewpoint automation cannot be objectively assessed. However, at least qualitatively, the experimental results referred above clearly suggest that autonomous robotic camera assistance in MIS has a realistic chance to

- improve the endoscopic view (positioning, image stability, independence from available camera assistant)

- reduce the OR staff required for simple laparoscopic interventions and free the assistants for other tasks in complex ones

- allow the surgeon to focus on his main tasks, without increasing his cognitive load for camera control.

At the same time, there are two issues with current approaches. They are either

- too constrained to represent the minute differences in positioning required for an optimal view or

- require extensive manual modeling of know-how for each surgical task in each intervention type.

Table 2.2: Overview of previous approach on automation of endoscope positioning. The number under class corresponds to those in Fig. 2.39. "VS" stands for Visual Servoing.

Year	Authors	Robot	Class	Method	Ref.
1994	Lee and Uecker et al.	AESOP (2.1.2)	1	Markerless VS	[177], [178], [179]
1996	Casals et al.		6	Task-dependent VS modes	[209], [210]
1996	Wang et al.	AESOP (2.1.2)	8	Action sequences with VS	[215], [216]
1997	Wei and Omote et al.	AESOP (2.1.2)	3	VS with color markers with explicit rules	[196], [194], [195], [197]
1998	Kudo et al.		1	VS with color markers	[180]
2001	Nishikawa et al.	Custom (cf. LARS 2.1.4)	3	Face control	[198], [199], [200], [201]
2002	Zhang et al.	Custom	1	VS with mono-chrome markers	[181]
2004	Ko and Kwon et al.	KaLAR	8	Step-dependent voice or VS with color markers	[217], [218], [219]

2006	Nishikawa et al.	Custom (cf. LARS 2.1.4)	6	VS with pre-operatively defined zoom ratio	[211]
2006	Sivadasan	AESOP (2.1.2)	1	Eye gaze; Joystick	[182]
2006	Voros et al.	ViKY (2.1.9)	3	Markerless VS with 3D from geometry	[202], [203]
2007	Bourger et al.	AESOP (2.1.2)	1	Model-free VS	[183]
2008	Nishikawa et al.	Custom (cf. LARS 2.1.4)	5	VS with learned angle-distance relation	[212]
2009	Polski et al.	SOLO-ASSIST (2.1.11)	1	Electromagnetic servoing	[185]
2010	Munduri	ZEUS (2.1.23)	3	Kinematics-based servoing	[204]
2010	Noonan et al.	Custom	1	Gaze control	[188]
2010	Osa et al.	Endo[PA]R	1	VS with color markers	[186]
2011	Weede et al.	LWR IV; RX90	8	VS with instrument path prediction	[220], [221]
2012	Song et al.	(Webcam)	3	VS with color markers	[205]

2013	Bauer et al.	SOLO-ASSIST (2.1.11)	8	Step-dependent voice or VS with color markers	[222]
2013	King et al.	(Webcam)	1	VS with color markers	[189]
2013	Lie and Zhang et al.	CoBRA-Surge (2.1.23)	1	Gaze control	[190], [191]
2013	Yu et al.	Custom Telema-nipu-lator	3	Kinematics-based servoing	[206]
2013	Fujii et al.	KUKA LWR IV	3	Gaze gestures and control	[207]
2014	Agustinos et al.	ViKY (2.1.9)	6	Step-dependent VS modes with 3D from geometry	[214]
2014	Rivas-Blanco et al.	Barret WAM	6	Surgical-Action-dep. VS; Offset learning	[213]
2014	Zhao et al.	ViKY (2.1.9)	3	VS color markers & 3D from geometry	[208]
2015	Li et al.	CoBRA-Surge (2.1.23)	1	Fuzzy Gaze control	[193]

3 System Architecture and Conceptual Overview

After motorized endoscope holders and approaches to the automation of camera positioning were surveyed in the previous chapter, the architecture of the new method put forth in this thesis is described. Referring to the classification of viewpoint automation from section 2.2.2, the new approach can be characterized as context-aware, model-based planned (number 8 in Fig. 2.39).

This chapter is divided into two parts: First, the conceptual architecture of the knowledge-based cognitive system (cf. 1.3) that underlies this thesis (3.1). Second, the concrete mapping from the task of autonomous camera guidance to this conceptual framework (3.2).

3.1 Conceptual System Architecture

Fig. 3.1 shows the structure of knowledge-based cognitive *technical* systems as a block diagram.[1] There are two paths in this system. One path is about adding new information to the knowledge base (learning). The other paths utilizes the knowledge base for interpretation of the current scene and determining the next action (executing). The control flow in the system is cyclic: Information about environment and user is perceived by sensors. This raw data is then processed by interpretation algorithms that utilize different forms of encoded knowledge to infer relevant information about the current state. With

---

[1]In contrast to Fig. 1.11 interpretation and planning is treated in unison here. That is, the result of interpretation is not a description of the current state, but the course of action given the current state.

the help of further models from the knowledge base the next action is determined. The action is then executed and causes a change either in the environment or leads to new user input.

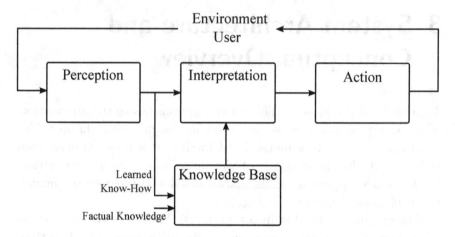

Figure 3.1: Conceptual architecture of a knowledge-based cognitive system.

Further details about each conceptual component are briefly discussed in the following sections. In order to make the presentation more vivid, a simple agent living in a two dimensional world will be used as an example (Fig. 3.2).

3.1.1 Perception

Perception refers to the ability of a system to acquire data about its environment.[2] Here environment is understood as some part of (simulated) physical reality, which behaves according to the laws of physics. In particular, objects have a position relative to some fixed global coordinate system. They can be influenced by external forces and have a certain appearance relative to surrounding illumination. Moreover, since only technical systems are considered here, perception

---

[2]The system is assumed to have access to its own state without requiring perception.

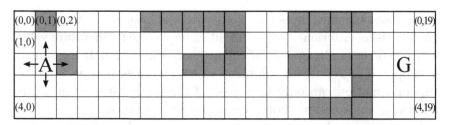

Figure 3.2: The agent A is used as an example throughout this section. Adjacent cells are specified by the neighborhood $\mathcal{N}$ of a cell (i,j): $\mathcal{N}_{(i,j)} = \{(i-1,j),(i+1,j),(i,j-1),(i,j+1)\}$, i.e. no diagonals. Agent A can distinguish between three states of adjacent cells: empty ($\square$), occupied ($\blacksquare$) and the goal G. The set of all empty cells is $\mathcal{E}$ and the set of all occupied cells is $\mathcal{O}$. Cells beyond the drawn ones are considered occupied. The agent's state $\mathcal{S}$ is fully determined by its current position p_t, i.e. $p_t = (2,1)$ here. Besides sensing neighboring cells, the agent can change his position to an empty adjacent cell, i.e. $p_{t+1} \in \mathcal{N}_{p_t} \cap \mathcal{E}$. The agents objective is to reach the goal G.

is accomplished by means of sensors. Each sensor captures certain data about the environment and is (sufficiently) robust or invariant to influences by other factors. For example, a camera acquires photometric data captured by its optical system from radiance in the field of view. At the same time, ambient temperature influences the data as well, but the latter is not *intended* to be measured by a camera. Thus it is assumed here that proper technical measures were taken to reduce the camera's sensitivity to all influences apart from scene illumination to the level of noise – at least under normal working conditions.

An important consideration here is what can still be considered sensor "raw data", i.e. where does perception stop and interpretation start. In case of a temperature sensor, a digital representation of the current temperature in degrees Celsius is perception data. A digital representation of the information "water is cooking" is considered outside the scope of sensor data. Whether the sensor requires information about circumstances that go beyond the measured quantity is a good decision criterion. In the current example, the temperature value will be correct independent of the measured material. If the sensor is supposed to report on the phase of a substance, here vaporizing, this information can only be correct if the temperature sensor has additional information about the measured substance.

For the example agent (Fig. 3.2), perception is a discrete value about the state of each cell in the neighborhood.

3.1.2 Interpretation

Interpretation is the two stage process of deducing information that is relevant to the system's objective from perception data and inferring a course of actions towards the objective. The first stage is often referred to as state estimation and the latter often called planning. Nevertheless, there are several classes of algorithms that do not allow a clear separation between these stages. Recent approaches for end-to-end learning (cf. [223]) with deep neural networks (DNNs) are a prime example of these. In this kind of end-to-end learning, raw perception data is feed directly into a neural network whose output is directly mapped to the motors of a robot. No layer in the DNN represents a clear separation between scene analysis and plan synthesis. Since the system in this thesis does not employ an end-to-end paradigm, but takes a more engineering oriented approach, at least a conceptual split in two stages is still useful here.

State Estimation

In state estimation perception data is interpreted to assess information about a state parameter that is relevant to the task but is not directly known as an output from perception. A camera image of an indoor scene showing a table and chairs does not provide information about tables and chairs before interpretation. Only after an object recognition and pose estimation algorithm processed the raw data is the information about table and chair positions accessible to the system. For the example agent, the ambiguity and uselessness of uninterpreted perception data is illustrated in Fig. 3.3.

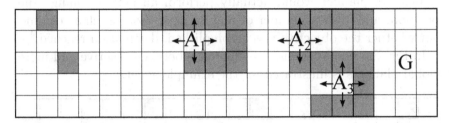

Figure 3.3: The current perception of agents A_1 and A_2 is identical. Obviously, A_1 can not make direct progress towards the goal G, while A_2 can. This information about the state is not directly contained in the perception of A_1 and A_2. The case for A_3 is not different if no assumption is made that the agents possess a memory of previous positions. Thus even in the simple example, perception is a necessary prerequisite, but without interpretation not much follows for the objective.

Planning

The output of planning is a feasible next step towards the system's objective given the current state information. A common example is path planning. Given a map of the environment[3], the (estimated) current position and a destination, the aim is to get from the current position to the destination. Depending on whether the planner is local or global, either a collision free next move towards the destination or a complete motion sequence from the current position to the destination is planned. The difference to purely reactive behavior that would not be considered planning is that a time interval instead of only the current point in time is taken into account. The planner in one form or the other simulates the situation that the immediate next step is taken and considers the resulting situation. Simulation can be as

---

[3]Commonly the map is two or three dimensional with binary or probabilistic occupancy information.

simple as virtually changing the current position in the occupancy grid and iterating this step to see whether the destination is reached. A reactive planner would actually perform an action, change the position, and after a number of real actions, position changes, find out whether the objective was accomplished, destination reached.[4]

In Fig. 3.4 planning and the difference between reactive and more global planners is illustrated for the example agent.

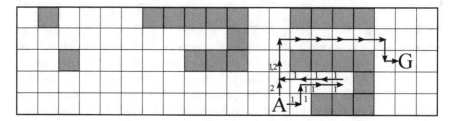

Figure 3.4: Assuming the coordinate of the goal G is known, a reactive planner with memory could work according to the following rule: If a free adjacent cell exists with a lower L_1 distance than the current position, move to it. Otherwise, backtrack to the last visited cell with an unvisited free adjacent cell and move there. The resulting behavior is exemplified by path 1. A global planner could employ the same procedure, however not as control rule, but as a search heuristic. Instead of actually moving along path 1, assuming this part of the map is already known, the planner would detect the dead-end and directly move upwards (path 2). Thereby, not only the next step is analyzed, but a time horizon, which leads to a better result in this case.

3.1.3 Knowledge Base

According to the paradigm of knowledge-based systems (cf. 1.3) a systems behavior should not only be determined by procedural programs,

---

[4]This results in an analogy between greedy algorithms and reactive behavior. Nonetheless, in both cases there are problems and problem instances where the computationally less expensive greedy/reactive process leads to an optimal solution.

but largely depend on declarative models. There are two advantages in utilizing a knowledge base instead of directly encoding the resulting task behavior: The first advantage is that more synergies can be exploited in the system. A procedural encoding has a single specific input-output behavior. Information or rather the relation between data elements encoded in declarative models can be easily combined with further models by algorithms working with these models as input data. For example, program P_1 computes the geometric center, i.e. the centroid $\mathcal{C}$, of a body b and program P_2 utilizes the center of mass $\mathcal{M}$ for physics simulation. Given a body with uniform density $\mathcal{U}$, the centroid is identical to the center of mass. This relation R can be easily encoded, e.g. in first order logic $\forall x : \mathcal{U}(x) \wedge \mathcal{C}(x, y) \rightarrow \mathcal{M}(x, y)$. However, usually a system that contains both P_1, P_2, R and the information that b is uniform $(\mathcal{U}(b))$ is not able to *automatically* compose all this information in order to run P_2 on b. If a model of the input data, output data and input-output relation of P_1 and P_2 is contained in a declarative model together with R and information about the instances, such as $\mathcal{U}(b)$, algorithms can be automatically compose a pipeline that first applies P_1 to b and infers that because of b's uniformity the output is suitable as input for P_2. The second advantage is a practical consideration. Instead of having to modify program code for each change in environment or task objective, a more general program can be written once and the environment-specific or task-specific aspects can be stored in models that are read as data.

It is useful to distinguish between two kinds of information in the knowledge base: encoded factual knowledge and models of learned know-how.

Modeling Factual Knowledge

The main criterion to distinguish between factual knowledge and know-how is that the former can be written down by a domain expert. The manually created model is sufficiently rich, comprehensive and accurate that expert judgement can be substituted algorithmically using only the model and information about the prior expressed in terms of the model. A prime example are mathematical formulas. Given a formula such as $f(x) = x^2$ and a model of the rules of calculus, more specifically the rules for symbolic differentiation, no further information or human input is required to derive the result $f'(x) = 2x$. Factual knowledge is not required to be deterministic or symbolic as long as it is known independently from creation of the model.

A prime example of factual knowledge in form of symbolic rule sets is illustrated in Fig. 3.5.

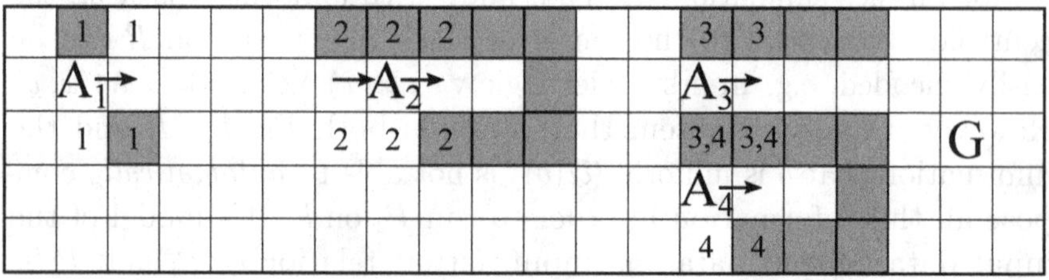

Figure 3.5: Assuming domain knowledge is available, for example: All dead-ends in the map start with an occupied cell above and an empty cell below followed to the right by an occupied cell above and an empty cell below. These dead-end detection rules could be stored in the knowledge base and added, removed or changed for each map without alternation to the agent program. Agent A_2 and A_4 would be able to detect the upcoming dead-end and stop moving in the current direction immediately. A_1 and A_3 would continue, but have to remember the just observed upper and lower cell while moving. The required memory length can also be derived from the rule set and thus coded universally.

Learning Know-How

Know-how is considered to be tacit knowledge. It is often related to the skills a person posses, which cannot be easily transfered by means of explicit communication such as natural language, mathematical models or program code. The most obvious example are motor skills. Some aspects of these are accessible by introspection, e.g. handwriting is largely performed by fingers and wrist, however, they cannot be easily put in physical units, e.g. the amount of force exerted between pen and paper in Newton or the momentary pen angle in degrees. Even if the requirement of introspectability is dropped and the information may be assessed experimentally, often basic statistic measures, e.g. mean and variance of a normal distribution, do not suffice to adequately capture the skill execution. Therefore machine learning is employed to fit the parameters of high-dimensional models or even create non-parametric models that are able to describe the complex (physical) relations that make up the skill. In other words, the learned model is not an encoding of a previously existing description, but creates the description in the first place.

How recordings of previous instances can be utilized as learned know-how is shown in Fig. 3.6 for the example agent.

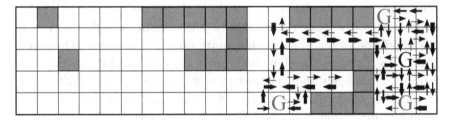

Figure 3.6: After a number of episodes in the same map, but with different unknown goal positions the example agent has recorded statistics on his previous actions. The arrow width indicates how often a move was part of a path that reached a goal *G*. Making the assumption that future goal locations are correlated with previous ones, the history can be used as a heuristic that guides the agent's future actions. For example in situations without further information, the agent could prefer to move into the directions that had a higher probability to reach the goal in previous episodes.

3.1.4 Action

Action refers to modification of the external environment's state or providing information to the user. For this thesis "embodied"[5] agents are the only relevant kind, that is agents whose environment is (a simulation of) the physical world. Therefore, an action must have a relevant *physical* influence on the system's environment. Even though the macrophysical world is treated as continuous in both space and time, it is often beneficial to distinguish between discrete and continuous actions. Continuous actions are commonly represented by a vector of real numbers, for example the two dimensional position of an object on a plane. Discrete actions on the other hand are based on a number of equivalence classes. These discretize a continuous state space into subregions whose inner structure is considered to be irrelevant. An example is the grid of the example agent (Fig. 3.2), which assumes that there is only one possible position within each cell or the exact position within the cell can be disregarded. The number of equivalence classes can be either finite or infinite. A grid discretization of a surface with a finite area is also finite. The same grid discretization of a plane is infinite. Actions can be also finite or infinite. If an agent can teleport to any position on an infinite grid, the number of actions can be considered infinite. However, given the same infinite grid and an agent that can only move to a finite number of adjacent cells, the actions are finite.

The actions of the example agent are discrete and finite, i.e. moving to a free adjacent cell.

---

[5]For more details on this concept, see chapter 2 in the book by Pfeifer and Bongard [224].

3.2 Camera Guidance as a Knowledge-based Cognitive System

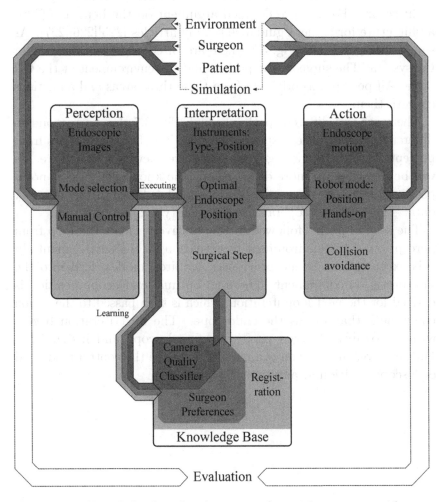

Figure 3.7: Knowledge-based architecture of cognitive camera guidance.

Having introduced the abstract concepts behind knowledge-based cognitive systems and illustrated with examples outside of robotics and surgery, this section shows how the autonomous camera guidance discussed in this thesis is mapped to a knowledge-based cognitive architecture. For a more detailed argument on the benefits of this architecture for camera guidance see my articles [225][226][227]. As shown in Fig. 3.7 and Fig. 3.8, there are three important entities for the system: The surgeon, the patient and the environment at the OR table. All perceptions originate from these three areas and all actions concern them.

There are two different paths through Fig. 3.7 that correspond to different phases in the system's lifecycle. The first path[6] goes from perception to the knowledge base and stores new elements there. As will be described in more detail below, the knowledge base is not a passive component, but actively trains models based on the new raw data. This occurs preoperatively for each type of intervention.

The second path[7], followed intraoperatively, closes the loop from perception of the environment to actuation on the environment. In this execution mode the previously acquired models feed into the interpretation component. There an optimal endoscope position is derived for the next loop iteration, which is then passed to the action component that moves the endoscope. The next iteration begins with a possibly changed positions of endoscope and instruments. Furthermore, the surgeon can manually change the control mode and endoscope position at any time.

---

[6]Corresponding to chapter 5.
[7]Corresponding to chapter 6.

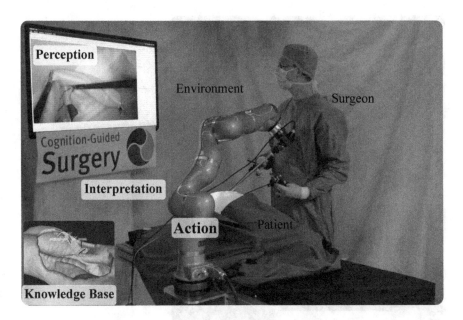

Figure 3.8: One concrete realisation of the cognitive camera guidance and its knowledge-based architecture: Laparoscopic rectal resection in the OpenHELP phantom with camera assistance provided by a lightweight robot.

3.2.1 Perception: Surgeon and Instruments

The first kind of perception data are the modalities available to the surgeon to manually change the behavior of the endoscope robot (Fig. 3.9). These comprise a foot pedal[8], voice commands, hands-on mode and web-based interfaces on touch devices, e.g. on a tablet or smartphone.

A major concern for automation of endoscope positioning is reliability. In terms of image processing or computer vision, endoscopic images pose several challenges: Smoke (Fig. 3.10a) caused by electrocautery, specular reflections due to the light originating from the

---

[8]The foot pedal is identical to the one used by the ViKY endoscope holder (2.1.9).

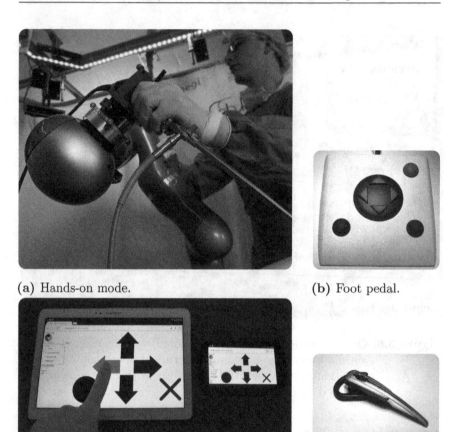

(a) Hands-on mode.   (b) Foot pedal.

(c) Web-based touch interfaces.   (d) Voice control.

Figure 3.9: Input modalities of the autonomous camera guidance.

endoscope and repetitive textures with a low contrast (Fig. 3.10b). A high amount of occlusion in the image because of the closeness between endoscope and scene objects. Furthermore, instead of dealing with rigid bodies, everything visible in an endoscopic image apart from the surgical instruments are deformable organs. Thus many object recognition approaches do not work well since they expect a fixed geometric relation between object features. This can be well seen in the contrast between the images in Fig. 3.10b and Fig. 3.10c that were taken only about 2 seconds apart.

There is progress in both hardware and image processing algorithms. Modern light sources are brighter and illuminate more uniformly, endoscopes are more light sensitive and have a higher resolution. Also, stereo laparoscopes are slowly gaining acceptance and open the possibility to transfer stereo vision methods to computer-assisted MIS (cf. [228]). Yet, segmentation and classification of abdominal organs from endoscopic images is still unreliable. For this reason, only the surgical instruments are tracked and their tip position is extracted from the endoscopic image (see 5.2.1).

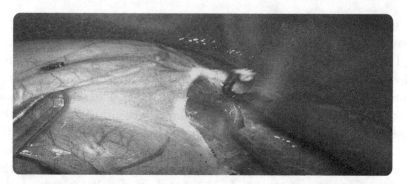

(a) Smoke caused by electrocautery.

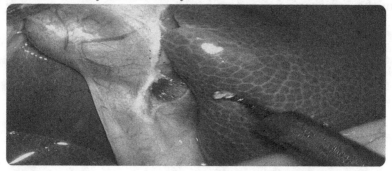

(b) Highly dynamic scene; specular reflections.

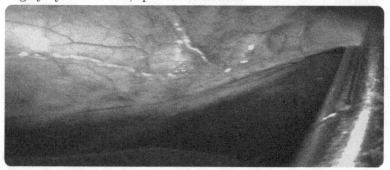

(c) Large deformations of soft bodies.

Figure 3.10: Three laparoscopic images extracted from a three second interval of laparoscopic cholecystectomy on a pig.

3.2.2 Interpretation: Optimal Endoscopic View

The core objective in this thesis is to provide the surgeon with an adequate endoscopic view throughout the intervention without a human camera assistant. Therefore the most relevant part of the system state is made up of the surgical actions and the surgeon's intentions regarding endoscope positioning. Given this information the interpretation component has to determine the next endoscope motion that is realized by the endoscope robot.

State Estimation: Intentions and Instrument Tips

Instrument tip position can be either directly acquired by external marker-based tracking or markerless from the endoscopic images by means of image processing. These different realizations of perception pipeline can be used interchangeably due to the modular platform on which the system is built (see chapter 4).

The surgeon's intentions and preferences to endoscope positioning are factored in the system's autonomous actions in three ways:

- Direct commands through the system's multimodal interfaces (cf. Fig. 3.9).

- Generic preferences and user profile settings, e.g. relative zoom and motion speed.

- Surgeon specific adaption of the positioning behavior over the course of multiple interventions.

These are further discussed in section 6.2.3.

Planning: Endoscope Positioning

There are five factors that influence the next endoscope position passed to the robot:

- Textbook knowledge about proper endoscope positioning stored in the knowledge base (3.2.3).

- The camera quality classifier from the knowledge base that determines optimal endoscope positions for the current situation (3.2.3).

- The adaptive sampling and fusion strategy for the camera quality classifier.

- Time decaying motion hysteresis (cf. Fig. 2.41) to steady the camera position.

- A motion model of the endoscope and robot that specifies the maximal scope of motion and the desired motion velocities (3.2.4).

Fig. 3.11 shows a block diagram of these elements. Details about the concrete interaction between these factors are given in section 6.2.2.

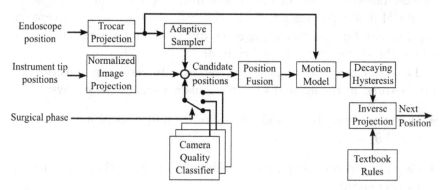

Figure 3.11: Block diagram of elements determining endoscope positioning.

3.2.3 Knowledge Base: Camera Quality Classifier

The knowledge base comprises factual knowledge and learned know-how. Factual knowledge pertains to (textbook) endoscope guidance rules, quality criteria for endoscopic views and a simple model of the surgical workflow. The learned models of proper endoscope positioning acquired by analysis of recorded interventions represent know-how from a human camera assistant.

Modeling Factual Knowledge: Textbook Endoscope Guidance

There are a few explicit rules about endoscope assistance that can be directly encoded in logic or formulas. One important rule is maintaining a stable image horizon, i.e. keeping the horizontal image axis parallel to the floor. Another is to avoid staining of the endoscope optics by contact with tissue.

Another set of factual knowledge relates to quality criteria of proper endoscope views. These present formalized criteria for assessment and annotation of endoscope positioning as good, neutral and poor. However, the rules are encoded in natural language and a surgical expert is required to annotate images with these labels. The reason is that the criteria cannot be generalized to simple rules, such as the instrument must be in a certain region with a certain distance (cf. Fig. 5.2 in chapter 5).

In order to reduce the complexity of the spatial learning problem, as described below, a formal model of the surgical workflow exists for each intervention type. The model partitions an intervention into surgical phases, steps and task (Fig. 3.12). Together with online phase recognition (5.2.2) the learned model can be trained separately for each phase or step and switched intraoperatively.

Learning Know-How: Spatial Relations

Without going into much detail, as will be done in chapter 5, a short summary of learning spatial know-how is provided here. The spatial relation between instruments and endoscope is what a good human camera assistant is capable of getting right. The approach put forth in this thesis, is to encode the spatial know-how in a model and use it for automated camera positioning. To this end, several interventions of the same type are recorded and annotated with a label how well the endoscope was positioned. A ternary classification in "good", "neutral" and "poor" endoscopic view was chosen. Of course, this process has a subjective aspect to it. Nevertheless, some assistants provide good camera assistance based on their ability to asses the

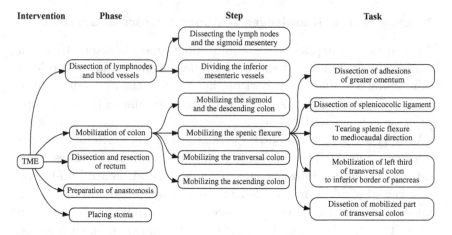

Figure 3.12: Excerpt of the workflow for laparoscopic rectal resection with total mesorectal excisions (TME) employed in the phantom evaluation (Ch. 7).

situation. Exactly this (subjective) tacit knowledge is to be captured in the model.

The model is formulated as a classifier. Given the endoscope and instrument positions in a specific encoding as input, the classifier's output is the ternary suitability of the camera view. Therefore, this classifier is termed camera quality classifier (CQC). The task is to *find* a good endoscope position, which the camera quality classifier does not directly provide as output.[9] Adaptive sampling over possible endoscope positions is used to answer the question what endoscope positions provide a good view given the current instrument positions. Fig. 3.13 shows the results of querying a CQC for a recorded point in time of a phantom experiment. The endoscopic view of the situation is shown in Fig. 3.13c together with a screenshot of the reconstructed 3D scene in Fig. 3.13d. The two upper images in the figure, show two different sampling strategies for the classifier: a fixed grid sampling

---

[9]A different formulation of the model using regression instead of classification is less suited because there are often several clusters of good poses. This multivariate distribution can be naturally comprised by the classifier formulation.

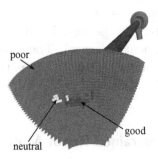

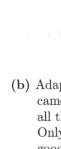

(a) Grid sampling the camera quality classifier at a fixed insertion depth around current endoscope pose for given instrument positions.

(b) Adaptive sampling of the camera quality classifier in all three degrees of freedom. Only positions evaluated as good are shown.

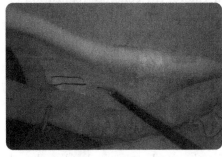

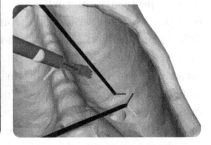

(c) Recorded endoscopic view of an intraoperative situation for which the camera quality classifier is queried.

(d) Virtual scene reconstructed from recorded data with actual and good candidate poses.

Figure 3.13: Illustration of the camera quality classifier. Endoscope poses are indicated by different arrows for good, neutral and poor positions.

and adaptive sampling. Only positions evaluated as good by the CQC are drawn in Fig. 3.13b to reduce occlusions. A more in depth analysis of Fig. 3.13a, by means of the virtual endoscopic view, shows that the area of good positions has both instruments in the field of view. The smaller area of neutral positions centers on the right instrument (scissors) without showing the left instrument (grasper). The latter situation is quite common in earlier steps of the recorded data as the grasper is only holding and tensioning the colon, but not of further interest while static.

3.2.4 Action: Smooth and Pivot-constrained Robot Motion

The component most closely tied to classical robotics is the action component. Here the repositioning of the endoscope is accomplished in physical reality. Not only geometry and kinematics, but also dynamics have to be accounted for. In minimally-invasive surgery one additional concern is to maintain the trocar point as invariant point of the endoscope motion (cf. Fig. 1.10). Furthermore, the concrete realization of endoscope positioning with the special constraints at the OR table is important, as can be seen from the large amount of literature on different motorized endoscope holders (cf. 2.1). Therefore, it should be possible to evaluate the automated camera guidance approach presented here with robots featuring different kinematics. To separate camera positioning algorithms from realization of endoscope motion, a proper layer of abstraction was incorporated into the modular research platform that is described in the following chapter. In the context of this thesis, control and interfaces for three robots were developed and utilized for autonomous camera guidance (Fig. 3.14).

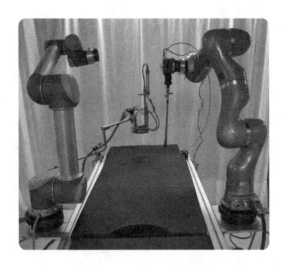

Figure 3.14: The three robots for which trocar-constrained collision free
motion was implemented in order to evaluate the unmodi-
fied camera guidance algorithm on them. From left to right:
Universal Robots UR5, Endocontrol ViKY and KUKA
LWR IV.

4 Modular Research Platform for Robot-Assisted Minimally-Invasive Surgery

4.1 The Robot Operating System (ROS)

The Robot Operating System (ROS) [229] is an open source middle-ware and a collection of associated software frameworks for modular (distributed) robot software. A focus of the middleware is exchange of streaming data[1] under soft real-time conditions while maintaining a high runtime flexibility. ROS is often used in a research context where heterogeneous software components, often developed in isolation by different people, must work together across multiple computers. Interoperability is ensured by common network message formats, native client libraries for several programming languages (i.a. C++, Python, Matlab, Android, Lisp) and protocol gateways, e.g. JSON over Web-Sockets. A large number of ROS-wrappers for other large software frameworks such as OpenCV[2], PCL[3] and OMPL[4] are available. There are also drivers for many common sensors, actuators, devices and whole robots available. Furthermore, advanced functionality such as simultaneous localization and mapping (SLAM)[5] and collision free path planning[6] are well integrated with ROS. One big advantage of

---

[1] The most common use cases assume a fast local network, like Gigabit Ethernet, and message frequencies of up to 1 kHz.

[2] http://opencv.org

[3] http://pointclouds.org

[4] http://ompl.kavrakilab.org

[5] See the navigation stack http://wiki.ros.org/navigation.

[6] See the MoveIt! http://moveit.ros.org/.

ROS compared with other middleware frameworks are the support tools such as 2D and 3D visualization[7] and introspection capabilities. The Gazebo robotics simulator[8] although usable independently of ROS is well integrated with ROS through plugins.

Processes that use the ROS middleware are called *nodes*. There are two basic communication mechanism implemented in ROS:

- *Services*: Synchronous request&response remote procedure calls (RPCs).

- *Topics*: Asynchronous unidirectional data streams modeled after the publish-subscribe pattern.

Both services and topics are strongly typed. The transported data types are called *messages* and defined in a special interface description language (IDL) from which native types for each programming language are generated. The *roscore*[9] acts as a well-known entry point with naming service and registry. If a node wants to call a service for the first time or subscribe to a topic, it contacts the roscore to receive the IP address and port of the other node (Fig. 4.1). The topic mechanism allows multiple publishers and multiple subscribers on the same topic. This is realized by means of multiple point to point connections.[10]

Actions built on top of services and topics, provide a communication pattern for long-running requests with intermediate feedback and preemption. A valuable in-depth article on the semantics of communication patterns in ROS and other robotic middleware systems was published by Schlegel et al. [230]. Apart from the means of communication, three further ROS components require a short introduction:

---

[7]Especially the feature-rich rviz tool http://wiki.ros.org/rviz.

[8]http://gazebosim.org

[9]Actually roscore is a collection of several nodes that act as central registry (ROS master), provide the parameter server and a central logging infrastructure (rosout).

[10]By default ROS uses TCP for all connections.

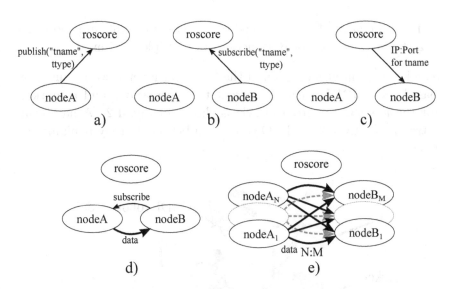

Figure 4.1: Interaction between ROS nodes and the roscore: A node announces the availability of a topic by notifying the roscore (a). In a similar manner, publishers announce themselves to the roscore (b). Once a (subscriber,publisher)-pair for the same topic is known to the roscore, the IP address and port of the respective publisher is handed to the subscriber (c). The subscriber node directly contacts the publisher node to initiate a direct data connection (d). The relation between subscribers and publishers on the same topic can be N:M (e).

- The *tf* package[11] maintains a time-variant coordinate transformation tree in a distributed manner [231].

- The Unified Robot Description Format (*URDF*)[12] is a file format used to model the visual, geometric, kinematic and dynamic properties of a robot with serial kinematics.

---

[11]http://wiki.ros.org/tf
[12]http://wiki.ros.org/urdf

- The *roslaunch*[13] file format and tool are used to configure and start a (hierarchical) set of ROS nodes (on multiple machines).

The live system visualization of the LWR during endoscope guidance based on a URDF with all current transformations and a marker for the medical phantom in rviz is shown in Fig. 4.2. A hands-on introduction to ROS and ROS tools can be found in my book article [232].

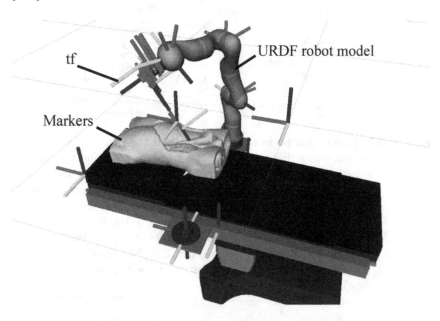

Figure 4.2: Rviz visualization of current coordinate transformations (tf) and robot state (URDF).

4.2 A Modular Platform

Evaluation of the knowledge-based camera guidance on different robots and with different sets of optional assistance functions was an

---

[13]http://wiki.ros.org/roslaunch

important goal for the thesis. Thus, instead of a direct coupling between perception, interpretation and action in a single program, reusable components were created.

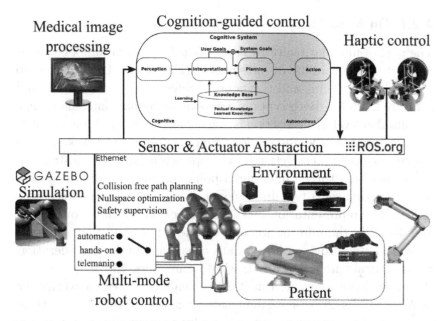

Figure 4.3: Overview of the modular platform for robot-assisted minimally-invasive surgery. Perception components include Kinect RGB-D cameras, Time-of-Flight cameras, endoscopic cameras, marker-based tracking systems, ultrasound and haptic input devices. Components to perform physical actions are two KUKA LWR IV, a Universal Robots UR5 and an Endocontrol ViKY. Each robot offers several control modes. Independent subsystems built on these components include a bimanual haptic telemanipulator and multiple RGB-D camera people tracking.

An overview of the hardware and software components that are integrated into a modular research platform for robot-assisted (minimally-invasive) surgery is shown in Fig. 4.3.[14] A description of the components and subsystems can be found in a book article published by myself together with several colleagues [233].

4.2.1 On Modularity

The goal of modular (software) systems is the separation of concerns and interchangeability of subsystems (Fig. 4.4). In the scenario at hand, subsystems and components refer to physical devices and software modules. Both types of components become interchangeable if a suitable level of abstraction is defined for their (core) functionality.

Unfortunately, the abstraction often depends on the task. For example, the proper abstraction for the tips of a laparoscopic instrument can either be a three dimensional point in some coordinate system or the (normalized) two dimensional coordinates in the endoscopic image. The representation must guarantee that all data sources are able to fill in the information and on the other hand that sufficient information is provided for all data consumers under consideration. If instruments are externally tracked by markers, the 3D position is the more obvious format. But if image analysis is used to extract the instrument tips, 2D seems a more natural choice. In this case the three dimensional representation was chosen due to requirements of the data consumers. If only a monoscopic laparoscope is used, the distance to the optics is approximated by the diameter of the instruments in the image. Together with the endoscope position, known through the robot kinematics, all data is available for the 3D representation. Another interface choice that required careful consideration is the endoscope position (see 5.3.2), because the robot have from as few as 3 degrees of freedom up to 7 DoFs (cf. Fig. 3.14). More observations

---

[14]The platform is a joint effort with several colleagues in the IAR-IPR at the KIT. My own contributions, beyond the cognition-guided camera control, include a comprehensive simulation infrastructure, ROS drivers and wrappers for the robots and endoscope cameras. These will be described in more detail here. Contributions of my colleagues are mentioned and references to more elaborate descriptions are provided.

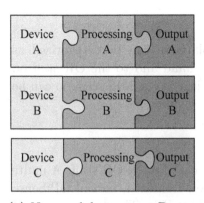

(a) Non-modular system: Parts are closely coupled, each connection between different parts is unique.

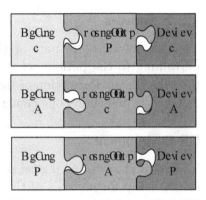

(b) In a non-modular system, parts cannot be rearranged without requiring modification.

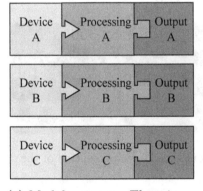

(c) Modular system: There is a well-defined interface for each functional type of a part.

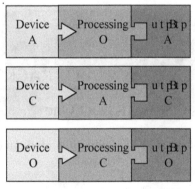

(d) In a modular system, parts can be rearranged to compose new functionality.

Figure 4.4: Illustration of how modular systems facilitate exchange of subsystems without inducing modifications in existing parts.

about modularity in robotics can be found in two co-authored papers [234][235].

4.2.2 Sensors

The sensors that are part of the platform can be categorized as pertaining to the patient on the one hand and to the OR staff on the other hand. Perception of the patient in the MIS scenario can be assigned to the endoscope camera.

OR Environment

In clinical practice, no digital sensors capture the OR staff. A multi-sensor setup for analysis of the OR environment, named OP:Sense [236], is part of the lab setup at the IAR-IPR. The ceiling-mounted sensors are four Microsoft Kinect 360, four Microsoft Kinect One, six PMD time-of-flight cameras and an ARTTRACK2 marker tracking system consisting of six capture devices (Fig. 4.5).

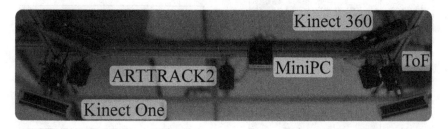

Figure 4.5: Ceiling-mounted environment sensors for perception of the OR staff.

Utilization of these sensors in order to improve safety and ergonomics in the OR is investigated in several research projects: Real-time collision avoidance for robot-assisted surgery [237], intuitive human-robot interaction in the OR [238] and people detection with multiple time-of-flight and Kinect cameras [239].

Endoscope

Two kinds of endoscope cameras are integrated into the system. The first is a medical endoscope camera, R. Wolf Endocam Logic HD (cf.

Fig. 1.3a), which is wired to a frame grabber device, Blackmagic Deck-Link 4K Extreme. The second camera type is the class of industrial cameras that provide network interface based on the GigE Vision standard, e.g. Allied Vision Manta G-201C. A custom ROS wrapper for each camera type converts the images into a common message format, which allows to use both cameras interchangeably. Tools from the ROS image_pipeline[15] are used to intrinsically calibrate and undistort the endoscopic images.

4.2.3 Distributed Processing

As explained above (4.1), ROS enables to transparently distribute robot software across multiple machines. This is utilized in the autonomous camera guidance system for two reasons: First, limited computational resources of single desktop machines. Second, to increase reusability, to create encapsulated subsystems and to facilitate parallel lab experiments. Figure 4.6 shows a subgraph[16] of the ROS computation graph that makes up the intraoperative camera guidance. Image processing is spread across a standard desktop computer and a server equipped with two powerful GPUs to enable processing of endoscope images at camera frame rates. The foot switch (cf. Fig. 3.9b) is connected to a low-power embedded system, Raspberry Pi, in order have a portable stand-alone system. Control of the LWR robots is performed on a dedicated machine with a real-time Linux kernel (see 4.2.4). Finally, the camera guidance algorithm, running on a desktop machine, as top-level control subscribes to information about instrument tips and the current endoscope position provided by the other machines. Since only the topic name is used to identify and connect to other components, the camera guidance node does not require information about deployment details. For example, given a sufficiently powerful machine, all components could be run on a single machine without changing a single line of code or configuration files.

---

[15]http://wiki.ros.org/image_proc
[16]Additional edges, such as those to and from the ubiquitous tf topic, have been removed from the node-induced subgraph.

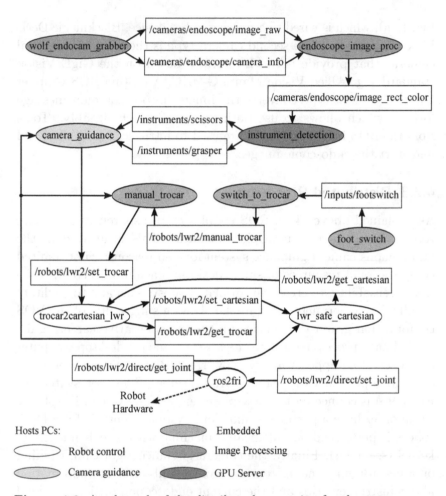

Figure 4.6: A subgraph of the distributed processing for the autonomous
camera guidance system. Nodes are drawn as ellipses and
topics as rectangles. The ellipse shading corresponds to
different hosts.

4.2.4 Actuators

Three different robots (see Fig. 3.14 in 3.2.4) have been integrated
into the platform for evaluation of automated endoscope positioning.

Their ROS interfaces and, more importantly, a common representation of all their aspects in the platform are described next.

KUKA LWR IV

The KUKA LWR IV has seven degrees of freedom and features torque sensors in each joint. External control is possible by means of network interface based on the UDP protocol, named Fast Research Interface (FRI). FRI allows control of the individual joints with a frequency of up to 1000 Hz. A special ROS node, ros2fri, that is divided into normal and real-time[17] threads bridges between ROS and the FRI protocol. This allows for reliable external control at 1 kHz. A separate ROS node, lwr_safe_cartesian, without strict real-time requirements provides Cartesian control on top of the joint topics. This node also performs collision checking with respect to the static environment, e.g. the OR table. The latter function is implemented with help of the MoveIt framework (cf. 4.1). A ROS action interface is provided by a generic node, trajectory_action2topic, that maps between action commands and the control topics just described.

Universal Robots UR5

The Universal Robots UR5 is a six degree of freedom lightweight manipulator. It can be externally interfaced by uploading an URScript program. Within the program, further network connections can be opened that allow to servo the joints with up to 125 Hz.

Based on the universal_robots driver[18] developed by the ROS Industrial Consortium[19], a ROS wrapper was developed that provides the same interfaces as the ones described above for the LWR. This provides a clean separation between high-level control and execution by a specific robot. Since different control concepts require access

---

[17]Using the Linux scheduling class SCHED_RR with priority 90 on a RT_PREEMPT kernel.
[18]http://wiki.ros.org/universal_robot
[19]http://rosindustrial.org

to different interfaces, e.g. trocar, Cartesian or joint coordinates, common interfaces were provided at multiple points in the control pipeline (Fig. 4.7). A controller implemented as a ROS node can use ROS mechanisms to query what parts of the interface are available. For example, the LWR provides a measurement of external torques, which the UR5 is lacking. If a node requires the torque measurement, it simply checks whether these are available and aborts otherwise, telling the user that the robot lacks a required capability. A node that only requires a subset of the robot's capabilities, for example position control, does not have to distinguish between the different robots and can use both interchangeably.

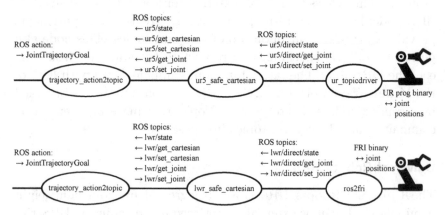

Figure 4.7: Unified ROS interfaces for the KUKA LWR IV (7 DoF, FRI interface) and the Universal Robots UR5 (6 DoF, URScript interface).

Endocontrol ViKY

The hardware of the ViKY endoscope holder has already been described in section 2.1.9. Here only the newly created external interface is summarized. ViKY does not provide any external interfaces by default. However, due to the use of a standard PC in ViKY's control box together with standard industrial motor drivers, it was possible to make ViKY externally controllable in software. Fortunately, the ViKY mainboard provides an Ethernet interface, which was used to connect it with ROS. Given ViKY's spherical 3 DoF kinematics, no Cartesian interface is provided, but one in joint and trocar coordinates (cf. 6.1.5).

4.2.5 Model Management

The modular platform comprises four robots r that can be attached in two places at the OR table p. Each robot can carry one out of about eight different tools t, each tooling using one of two connectors c. Thus there are up to^{20} $\frac{r!}{(r-p)!} \cdot \frac{t!}{(t-p)!} \cdot c = 112$ combinations. Since these contain many redundancies, e.g. same robots attached to same places, but with different tools, care must be taken that these are not simply plain copies of each other. The software engineering principles "Single Point of Truth" (SPOT) and "Don't repeat yourself" (DRY) demand that every information unit is only stored once. Since URDF is a flat XML format, this must be achieved by other means than URDFs native features. Therefore, a hierarchical scheme was employed that allows to include (partial) robot models into others. In this manner each fixed relation between items is stored exactly once (Fig. 4.8).

For historical reasons there are two description formats for robots in the ROS ecosystem, the dominant one being URDF (cf. 4.1). Yet, the Simulation Description Format (SDF) is the native model format of the Gazebo robotics simulator (cf. 4.3.1) and is more expressive than URDF, e.g. it can also deal with parallel kinematic chains. In order to avoid violation of the SPOT/DRY principle due to this issue, a converter tool, sdf2urdf[21] was developed that converts global link coordinate convention SDFs into joint local coordinate convention URDFs. Thus it is now possible to describe composite robots within the ROS ecosystem in a unified, hierarchical manner.

---

[20]Not all combinations of robots, places and tools are possible, e.g. the ViKY endoscope holder can only carry four different tools.
[21]`wiki.ros.org/sdf2urdf`

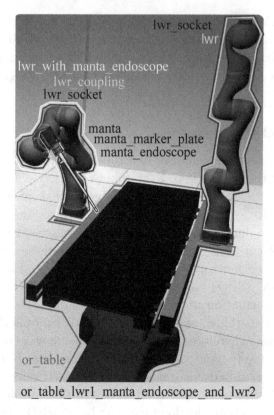

Figure 4.8: An illustration of the hierarchical composition of robot models.

4.3 Simulation Environment

Working with robot hardware is inevitable when investigating an autonomous endoscope guidance system. Simulations tend to be too orderly and deterministic, i.e. they do not capture the "messy" real world data. Furthermore, the system must be evaluated by surgeons in realistic scenarios. The more realistic the scenario, the higher the chance that research results will carry over in clinical practice. Having said this, in research and development an extensive simulation is invaluable, especially for an iterative research process. The simulation allows to quickly evaluate software changes without having to go through a tedious test cycle in the lab. Furthermore, software quality in robotics – even in a research setting – can be improved through a novel kind of testing methodology that I named Robot Unit Testing (see 4.3.3).

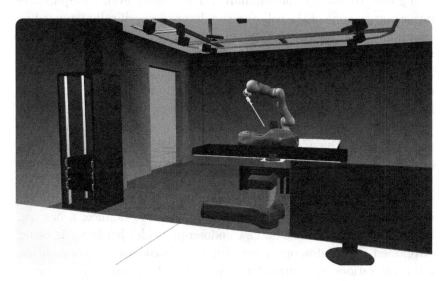

Figure 4.9: Screenshot from the comprehensive simulation environment for the knowledge-based camera system built on the Gazebo simulator.

In Fig. 4.9 a screenshot of the simulation environment for automated endoscope guidance is shown. It comprises simulation models of endoscopes, robots, surgical instruments, environment, environment sensors and the OpenHELP phantom (cf. 7.2.1). All devices of the modular platform that exist in simulation have the same interface as the real devices. Thus ROS nodes, such as the camera guidance one, can be run against the simulation without any modification or recompilation (cf. upper part of Fig. 3.7). In the remainder of this section the current state of robotics and surgical simulators is briefly discussed, followed by my robot unit testing methodology.

4.3.1 Robotics Simulators

There are currently four robotics simulators that provide the basic functionality required for simulation of all aspects covered by the endoscope guidance system: Gazebo[22], MORSE[23], Webots[24] and V-Rep[25]. Out of these only Gazebo and MORSE are fully open-source. Being able to modify the simulator, if necessary even core parts, is important as none of the robotics simulators is specifically intended or commonly used for the scenario of minimally-invasive surgery. Both Gazebo and MORSE natively support ROS which means two things: First, virtual sensors, such as color and depth cameras, provide their data in the respective middleware format. Second, the simulator state is accessible (and can be modified) using tools provided by the middleware. Because the Gazebo robotics simulator [240] has been adopted by the Open Source Robotics Foundation (OSRF)[26] and used for the DARPA Robotics Challenge (DRC) it is better integrated with ROS and more feature complete at the time of writing.

There are two challenges that have to be faced in order to enable an extended use of the robotics simulator for camera guidance: geometric and visual realism. Since no new endoscope holder hardware is being developed and endoscope positioning is a task with low velocities, low accelerations and without the requirement for force-based control schemes, realistic dynamics, i.e. physics simulation, are not important. To put it another way, for endoscope guidance dynamics can be largely delegated to the joint control level. If a robot provides a position controlled interface, dynamics must not be explicitly taken into account for this task in higher layers of control.

Geometric realism boils down to having access to good CAD models of all relevant objects or creating them oneself. The collision checking algorithms built into modern simulators are able to directly deal with

---

[22]http://gazebosim.org

[23]https://www.openrobots.org/wiki/morse

[24]https://www.cyberbotics.com

[25]http://www.coppeliarobotics.com

[26]The OSRF is the maintainer of ROS since the original company that developed ROS, Willow Garage, shutdown in 2013.

polygon meshes. These meshes can be automatically generated from
CAD models with the required amount of accuracy.

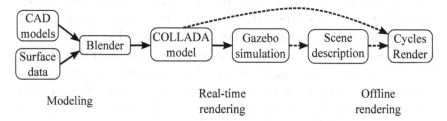

Figure 4.10: Integration of the Gazebo robotics simulator with the offline renderer Cycles. The Gazebo simulation triggers an
offline render process whenever a virtual sensor requests
high fidelity visual information. The physics engine usually
runs at 1 kHz, common cameras run at 30 Hz, thus even
if all camera frames are offline rendered only every 33rd
simulation step would require an offline pass, while all other
simulated sensors are served from the real-time engine.

Visual realism on the other hand is more difficult to achieve with current robotics simulators. Yet, it is important because the data provided
by the virtual (camera) sensors, such as the simulated endoscope, can
only be used with algorithms written for the real environment if it
is sufficiently realistic. In computer rendering there are two basic
approaches: Real-time[27] rendering and offline rendering. Without
going into detail here, real-time rendering usually employs rasterisa-
tion which directly maps the geometry of a virtual scene to pixels,
the most popular APIs being OpenGL and DirectX. Offline rendering
commonly refers to path tracing or ray tracing methods that follows
the path of light in the virtual scene to the pixels. Even though the
former is getting more powerful every year and adds more indirection,

---

[27]The term "real-time" here is not used in the same sense as in "real-time
systems". Real-time rendering refers to any procedure that is able to generate
computer graphics with at least roughly 30 frames per second (FPS). Real-time
systems refer to systems with time constraints, i.e. real-time systems do not only
provide logically correct results, but give guarantees that the results are given at a
specific time.

the latter method can still capture many more light phenomena such as global lightning effects and subsurface scattering[28].

Gazebo has a real-time rendering back end based on the OGRE engine[29] which uses OpenGL. Thus an effort was undertaken to improve the visual realism of Gazebo [242][241]. Fig. 4.11b shows some preliminary results for the medical phantom OpenHELP. Still a real-time rendering engine is not able to capture several of the visual aspects that occur in laparoscopic surgery. Therefore, a path was investigated that allows to seamlessly incorporate a raytracing engine into Gazebo. Of special concern was to have a single set of virtual objects in order to avoid inconsistencies as discussed above in section 4.2.5. The current solution works as follows (Fig. 4.10): COLLADA[30] is used as intermediate exchange format for visual models. Gazebo can directly import these models and use them for real-time visualization. In case more realistic visual data is required from a virtual sensor, the current state of the simulated environment is exported from Gazebo with reference to the COLLADA models. An offline renderer, Cycles Render, uses the information about the spatial composition of the object models and renders them under usage of the additional information contained in the object models. While the image is rendered Gazebo pauses the global simulation time. The rendered data (Fig. 4.11c) is then passed back to the virtual sensor in Gazebo, which thus provides a high fidelity image without slowing down the simulation all of the time.

---

[28]Subsurface scattering simulates how light is transported in translucent objects, such as human tissue.

[29]http://www.ogre3d.org

[30]An XML-based 3D asset exchange schema standardized by the Khronos Group.

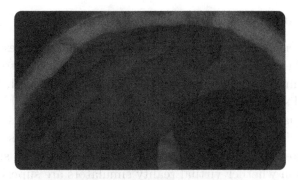

(a) Endoscopic image into the OpenHELP phantom.

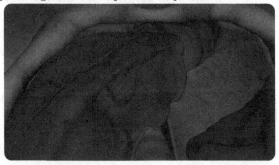

(b) Gazebo real-time rendering of a high fidelity OpenHELP model.

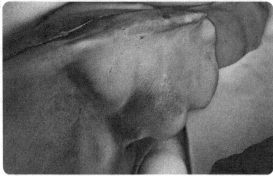

(c) Non real-time rendering of the OpenHELP model.

Figure 4.11: Visual realism in current robotics simulators and render engines (cf. [241]).

4.3.2 Laparoscopic Surgical Simulators

Having described how a *robotics* simulator is utilized for research into automated endoscope guidance, here a short comparison to the state of the art in laparoscopic *surgical* simulators is provided. A review on surgical simulation is available by Dunkin et al. [243] from 2007 and by Tanaka et al. [244] from 2015. From the systems described in these reviews, three systems are selected for a brief discussion on their features and what distinguishes them from robotics simulators. The question whether virtual reality simulators are superior to box trainers or complement them in surgical education is not posed here. The focus here is on technical features these simulators provide and how they could benefit simulation of robot camera assistance.

There are five basic validation aspects which are important to use simulators in surgical training [244]:

- Face: Experts judge the simulator to capture the relevant aspect realistically.

- Content: Experts judge the simulator appropriate for teaching purposes.

- Construct: The simulator is able to distinguish experts from novice surgeons.

- Concurrent: Correlation of simulation results with a gold standard.

- Predictive: Simulator can predict future performance of users.

Apart from these general considerations on validation of surgical simulators, an important question is to which purpose and surgical scenario the simulator can be applied. Two broad categories are simulators for conventional MIS and for robotic MIS, i.e. for the da Vinci robot (cf. 2.1.23). In contrast to open surgery MIS is always performed with an additional layer of indirection (cf. Fig. 1.4 in section 1.1.2). While this is a clear disadvantage of the minimally-invasive approach, it is an advantage for simulation purposes. It suffices to replicate the handles and trocar kinematics of laparoscopic instruments or the da Vinci input devices respectively. Since the operating site is viewed on a monitor in MIS, the difference when using a simulator does not become obvious in the modalities as would be the case for open surgery.

The LapSim simulator for laparoscopic surgery [245][246], Surgical Science Inc., exists in two versions. The portable version consists of two input devices that mimic the behavior of laparoscopic instruments inserted to the trocar, but without haptic feedback. For computation and visualization a normal desktop computer is employed. The other version consists of a console that provides two laparoscopic instruments handles with haptic feedback and an endoscope handle. LapSim offers training modules for basic skills, full procedures and endoscope positioning. Visualization is either a game-like training environment or a more realistic environment generated by real-time rendering.

The LAP Mentor [247], Simbionix, is also a trainer for laparoscopic surgery that exists in a portable and an integrated version. Again the portable device does not offer haptic feedback or endoscope control. Several different types of intervention from comparatively simple cholecystectomy to complex ones such as nephrectomy[31] can be selected. Visual realism is at the level of modern real-time game engines.

The da Vinci Skills Simulator (dVSS) [248], Intuitive Surgical, provides basic skill training with basic graphical visualization. As the simulator is a product of the da Vinci manufacturer the original surgical console is used. The dV-Trainer [249], Mimic Technologies Inc., mimics the console of the da Vinci in terms of input devices and display. Visual feedback does not aim for visual realism, but shows colorful game-like environments. The RoSS [250], Simulated Surgical Sciences LLC, also mimics the da Vinci's surgeon console. Visualization uses anatomical looking backgrounds, but the manipulation tasks employ simple colored objects. The Robotix Mentor [251], Simbionix, provides a compact surgeon console with freely moveable, i.e. not mechanically supported, input devices. Beyond basic skills,

---

[31]The surgical removal of a kidney.

also procedures can be trained in simulated anatomical surroundings with high visual realism. In all three simulators the da Vinci does not appear as a robot, which is not surprising, given that only the operating site is of interest.

The basic difference between robotics simulators, such as Gazebo, and laparoscopic surgical simulators is rigid body and soft body dynamic simulation. How closely the simulated soft bodies match the behavior of actual tissue has not been evaluated. However, videos of the soft body simulation suggest that especially the interaction with surgical tools is only a rough approximation. There is no fundamental difference between the employed rendering engines. Naturally, there are many differences with respect to what is built on top of the dynamics engine and the real-time rendering engine. For example, support for simulated sensors and actuated multibody systems, i.e. robots. Ideally, a surgical simulator could be extended to also simulate the surgical robot including the immediate surroundings at the OR table. For automated endoscope guidance, when disregarding the robot that positions the endoscope, current surgical simulators already provide all required functionality. At the same time, the visual realism would have to be evaluated not in terms of human perception, but for machine perception. A quality criteria is that computer vision algorithms which work with a certain quality[32] on real data q_r should ideally have the same quality when run on the simulated data q_s. Thus a metric for "computer perception realism" could simply be CPR $= 1 - |q_r - q_s|$, which becomes 1 if the quality is identical and becomes smaller with increasing difference between q_r and q_s.

4.3.3 Robot Unit Testing

I propose Robot Unit Testing (RUT) as a *methodology* for a new kind of unit tests specific to software-based systems that interact with their

---

[32]The measure of quality can be any criterion relevant for the algorithm, but is assumed to be normalized. For example in machine learning precision, recall or the F_β score would be good candidates. For segmentation the Dice coefficient could be employed.

physical environment A brief synopsis is given here, for further details
see my paper on the subject [252].

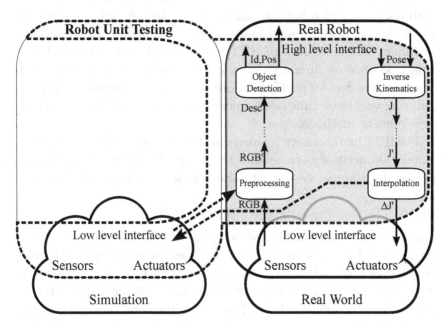

Figure 4.12: Robot unit testing utilizes all components in the shaded
area in the same manner as they are utilized on the real
system. The highest level interfaces are used to command
the robot and the lowest level interfaces are mapped to
and from simulation. Test coverage of individual units is
maximized and integration tests are performed at the same
time.

Robot unit testing is not about a specific technical solution, it is
about testing methodology (systematic analysis and best practices)
for robotics. Its main focus is to achieve a novel level of automated
test coverage for robots. A simulator substitutes the real environment
of the robot in terms of both perception input and action output
(Fig. 4.12). The robot software is required to allow rerouting of sensor
input and actuator output at start time, which is at least true for

ROS and others widely used robotic middleware systems. Writing RUTs often requires less effort to achieve good code coverage than conventional unit tests. The high-level interfaces are used to interact with the simulated robot. Simulation occurs by taking the commands at the lowest possible level and running them against a simulation instance. The drawback of RUT is the significantly increased test times because of simulation-in-the-loop testing. Fortunately, test cases can be run in parallel on one or multiple machines, thereby reducing wall clock time to an amount acceptable even for test-driven development methodologies.

The RUT methodology is based around a specific notion of *sufficient* simulation accuracy. Instead of requiring all relevant properties $\mathcal{P}$ holding for the real system r to also hold for the simulated system s, i.e.

$$\forall P \in \mathcal{P} : P(s) \leftrightarrow P(r)$$

a more continuous notion is developed. While this logical formula amounts to Leibniz's law[33] if all properties are considered, the principle never holds when comparing simulations to reality. Thus, this view does not provide any practical guidance. A more quantitative approach is thus chosen here: The overall distance between the real and simulated entity is defined over the properties, which also depends on the task t:

$$D = \sum_{P \in \mathcal{P}} d_{P,t}(s, r)$$

Each distance for a combination of property and task $d_{P,t}$, can then be observed in isolation to decide whether a given simulation is *sufficiently* realistic to use for testing.

For example, the geometric and kinematic model of the LWR is sufficiently realistic to simulate endoscope positioning tasks t_e, i.e. d_{kin,t_e} is below a threshold. The advantage of this notion shows when comparing the visual realism. Obviously, the pixelwise difference[34]

---

[33]More precisely to the indiscernibility of identicals $\forall x \forall y \; x = y \Rightarrow \forall P (P(x) \leftrightarrow P(y))$.

[34]Calculated for example by Sum of Absolute Differences (SAD) or Sum of Squared Differences (SSD).

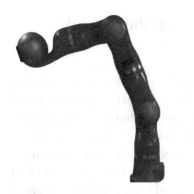 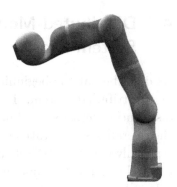

(a) Picture of real robot. (b) Simulation of robot.

Figure 4.13: Comparison of real and simulated KUKA LWR IV.

between Fig. 4.13a and Fig. 4.13b is quite large (Fig. 4.14a). Put in different terms, $d_{\mathrm{vis,SSD}}$ is going to be high. Yet, the same model has a much higher grade of visual realism, if the algorithm to be tested utilizes other features such as edges[35] (Fig. 4.14b), i.e. $d_{\mathrm{vis,edge}} \ll d_{\mathrm{vis,SSD}}$.

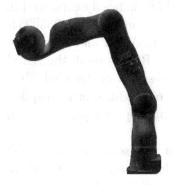 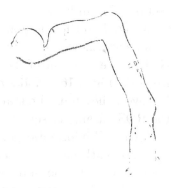

(a) Pixelwise absolute difference.

(b) Edge differences.

Figure 4.14: Visual differences of Fig. 4.13 compared by two measures.

---

[35]For example computed by Sobel operators.

4.4 Distributed Monitoring, Reliability and System Diagnosis

As described at the beginning of this chapter, ROS is a very flexible and distributed system. The combination of runtime flexibility and distribution across several machines can make it hard to reason about the overall system status or to find the source of an error. This is especially true for a lab setting, which is concurrently used by multiple researchers. For example, if one researcher works on the perception side only and another one on the action side, they might not share any single component. Yet, due to using the same set of hosts and common network infrastructure, crosstalk could occur even in this situation. A much more common situation is that also nodes are shared in the lab. As explained above (cf. Fig. 4.1), each additional subscriber increases the network load.

To deal with issues that can arise in the modular platform, Advanced ROS Network Introspection (ARNI) was created by myself together with a group of undergraduate students. How ARNI increases the reliability and introspectability of the platform on which the knowledge-based camera guidance is built is briefly explained in section. For an in depth account on ARNI see my articles [253][254].

In Fig. 4.15 the components that make up ARNI and their interactions are shown. If a current version[36] of ROS is used, the ARNI GUI can be used out-of-the-box to get an overview of the whole ROS network (Fig. 4.16). Nodes do not need to be modified or recompiled, however, they must be started after setting a special parameter on the ROS parameter server.

Having all information in one place is only possible because ARNI builds on gathering and analysis of *metadata* instead of the payload data. No single computer can handle aggregating all data streams in large ROS networks such as the modular platform presented in this chapter. Yet, even a host with low processing power can handle to aggregate the metadata of all network streams, such as frequency,

---

[36]ROS Indigo or later.

bandwidth, latency, jitter and dropped messages. The amount of bandwidth requires to describe data streams is small and independent of the payload bandwidth. Information about individual connections is further summarized at the topic level.

In some cases, problems that become visible at the level of ROS connections, e.g. dropped messages or high latencies, originate in over-loaded host computers. Therefore, ARNI can also collect information about each host and node. The information includes CPU, RAM and GPU usage, I/O statistics and transport layer bandwidth per node and aggregated per host. Furthermore, computer health information such as temperatures and disk utilization are published.

Given the metadata, the ROS network can be augmented by certain self-X properties through the definition of reference specifications. A specifications can state an interval for any property of a host, node, topic or connection that the property should adhere to at all times. For instance, one can specify an allowed interval for topic latency or the maximum allowed CPU temperature for a host. It is possible to have any number of partial specifications for subsystems – as long as they are not contradictory. These can be conveniently loaded during the start of nodes through roslaunch.

The final part of the ARNI system is the countermeasure node that can automatically act on the deviation of the system from its specification. Based on the rated metadata, the countermeasure node checks Boolean formulas and runs a user defined action if a formula is satisfied. Countermeasures can be run on any host that runs the ARNI host interface node. Similar to the specification format, countermeasures can be loaded and unloaded in parts.

A few basic specifications and countermeasures have been defined for the perception and action components of the camera guidance systems. Furthermore, ARNI is often utilized as a comprehensive dashboard during development to pin down bottlenecks or errors in the system.

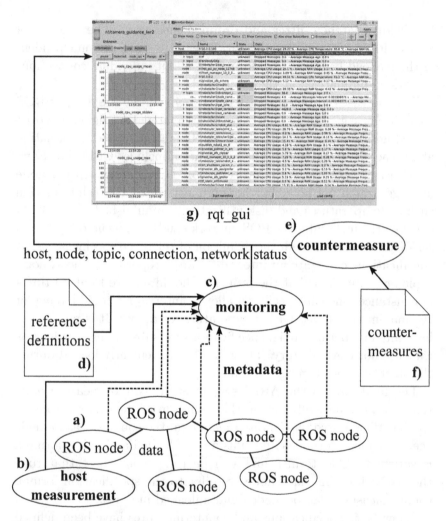

Figure 4.15: Overview of ARNI: a) Publishing of connection statistics
information; b) Publishing of information about hosts and
nodes; c) Comparison of current values to specification (d)
and publishing of rated statistics; e) Automatic execution
of given countermeasures (f) on deviation from specification; g) GUI which aggregates and displays information
from (a-c).

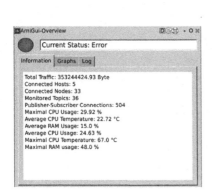

(a) ARNI Overview: Health state and aggregated information for whole network.

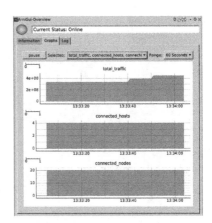

(b) ARNI Overview: Visualization of aggregated time series data.

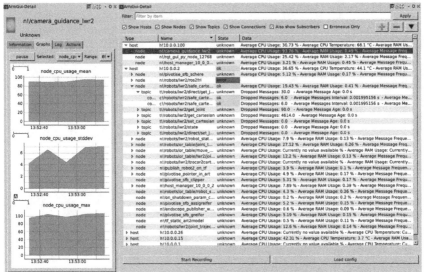

(c) ARNI Detail: The whole ROS network (hosts, nodes, topics and connections) at one glance. For each item that has specifications attached to it, the current health status is shown. All data is available in textual and plotted form.

Figure 4.16: Screenshots of the ARNI rqt GUI.

5 Learning of Surgical Know-How by Models of Spatial Relations

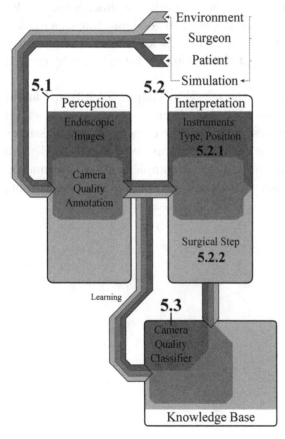

Figure 5.1: Overview of chapter 5 (cf. Fig. 3.7 p. 113).

The optimal spatial relation between instruments and endoscope is not a static one. It changes with the surgical task and the anatomical structures that are manipulated (Fig. 5.2). Even the optimal distance of endoscope to instruments varies widely, in relation to the optimal visual zoom of the operating site. As Nishikawa et al. [212] state: "The best zooming ratio depends on both the surgical procedure/phase and the habits/preferences of the operating surgeon." Defining these relations by hand is impractical for two reasons: First, there is often only a minute spatial difference between optimal and much less suited views, especially, when regarded over a period of time. Second, a lot of this information is not available, even to good assistants, as explicit knowledge, but only in the form of implicit know-how. Thus defining the optimal context-aware spatial relation by a list of manually created rules is infeasible.

Therefore, as outlined in the overview chapter (3.2.3), a learned model of camera guidance know-how is employed in the presented approach. This chapter describes how the camera quality classifiers that capture the assistant's know-how are modeled and learned. Also see my publications on the subject as complementary information [255][256]. For a recent survey on the general use of machine learning in surgical robotics, see the article by Kassahun et al. [26].

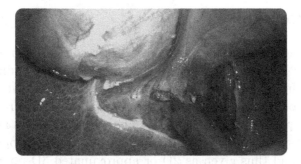

(a) A single instrument is centered in the image with high zoom. Note that two instruments are in use, the other one is holding up the gallbladder, but it is not required to be visible during dissection.

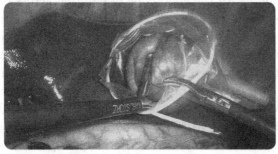

(b) Both instruments are in a central image position and equally important to the current task.

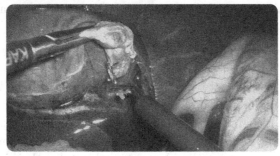

(c) Two instruments are visible, however the electrocautery in the center is the dominant one.

Figure 5.2: Illustration of the dynamic relationship between optimal endoscope position and surgical instruments in a cholecystectomy on a pig.

5.1 Perception

The data required for learning consists of recorded laparoscopic interventions and expert annotations. Intervention recordings must comprise the endoscope position and either externally tracked instruments or the endoscopic images. As in the intraoperative case, instrument positions are thereby given either as 3D points in a global coordinate system or they are extracted from the endoscopic images (see 5.2.1) and thus given as 2D or approximated 3D points in the endoscope frame. A registration between endoscope and patient is required with respect to orientation, i.e. the abdominal quadrants must correspond with the endoscope orientation across data sets.

Two types of annotations are required: Workflow information and camera quality. The workflow subdivides the whole procedure into multiple coarse surgical steps (cf. Fig. 3.12). Each step corresponds to a separate activity, concerns a particular anatomical structure and closely correlates with distinct instrument trajectories. If the recording contains all information required for a particular (online) phase recognition system (5.2.2), the annotation can occur (semi-)automatically. Annotation of the camera quality must be manually performed by an expert, since the very goal here is to capture the notion of optimal endoscope positioning in a model for the first time. Camera quality is encoded as a ternary value: good, neutral and poor.

5.2 Interpretation

This section describes two important components of the knowledge-based camera guidance system: Markerless instrument tracking and online phase recognition. While these are not research topics here in themselves, they are discussed because their current capabilities must be understood in order to build a system that takes their inaccuracies and errors into account. Furthermore, both components must be realized for evaluation of the system in phantom and animal studies (see chapter 7).

5.2.1 Tracking of Instrument Tips

In this section a brief summary of approaches for markerless instrument tracking is provided. This is done for two reasons: First, to substantiate the argument made in section 3.2.1 that instrument tip position is a good and reliable feature available without changes or augmentation of surgical instruments. Second, to classify the markerless instrument approach that has been integrated in the system. It is not the intention of this section to provide a comprehensive list of approaches, but to illustrate the range of different computer vision algorithms that have been applied to the task and give an idea how successful they are.

Uecker et al. (1995) [178] use pixelwise color classification with a Bayesian classifier as first step in their pipeline. After noise removal (median filtering), connected regions are segmented and labels are assigned to them. By means of shape analysis (centroid and moments, bounding box/trapezoid) areas with an instrument color signature but irregular shapes are discarded. Tracking over time is performed by predicting the segment position in the next frame and propagate the labels to these positions. An error of 5% of the image size is reported in four short ($\leq$ 35 frames) image sequences.

Climent et al. (2004) [257] extract edges from smoothed grayscale images and detect dominant straight lines in these by the Hough transform. A heuristic filter (minimum line length, start on image boundary) is employed to extract candidate lines. The end of the lines are used as instrument tip candidates. A first order model (velocities) is used to predict the next tip position. The tip with the smallest distance to the previous prediction according to a metric over the Hough table is selected as tip. The authors report that with tracking the detection is correct to 99% on a 128 image test sequence. At the same time systematic false detections are described (tool close to image edge, low contrast, fast instrument motions).

Doignon et al. (2005) [258] base their pixel-wise segmentation on a notion of color purity (color hue saturation feature). Instrument tips are assumed to be gray. Noise removal is performed by a cumulative histogram of absolute gradient values (a sigma filter approximation). Region segmentation is performed by region growing, using the hue saturation feature as homogeneity criterion, seeded on gray pixels at the image borders. Regions are classified by a closed contour representation with Fourier descriptors. Another classification proposed is based on intensity distribution moments. The moments are also used to determine the instruments principal axis. No results are reported in the publication.

Kim et al. (2005) [259] present a two-stage CONDENSATION[1] algorithm with a modified adaptive color model that is more robust to sudden changes in illumination of the tracked object. The first stage tracks the instrument shaft and extracts the tip region by fitting a line with weighted least squares to the shaft pixels. Along the instrument axis the instrument width is calculated. Using this information the second stage CONDENSATION algorithm is seeded in a rectangle around the tip region. No statistical results are reported.

Speidel et al. (2006) [260][261] use a Bayesian classifier for pixelwise color classification. The resulting image is median filtered. For tracking the CONDENSATION algorithm is used on the segmented image. An evaluation on 100 individual frames showed that the error was less than 4 pixels 82% of the time and in 93% less than 7 pixels for a resolution of 768 × 576

Voros et al. (2006) [202][203] use a geometric method based on measuring the position of the instrument trocars. The geometric aspects of the method have already been described together with the automated camera positioning approach in section 2.2 (p. 90). Using the known projection of the trocar point on the image plane P, dominant straight lines originating from P are extracted from the images by a Hough transform. The tip is then located along the instrument's axis by thresholding on color information. In an image sequence of less than 100 frames, 70% of the time the error was less than 5 pixels and to 87% less than 11 pixels. Yet, there were several

---

[1]Conditional Density Propagation.

wrong detections (lack of contrast, specular reflections) leading to very large errors.

Wolf et al. (2011) [262] extend the work by Voros et al. and use the CONDENSATION algorithm for tracking. They report a mean error of 27.8 px for 768 × 576 images over a 1050 frame sequence.

Allan et al. (2013) [263] use random forests with different color spaces as features for pixel classification. The largest connected region of instrument pixels is then segmented. Based on the moments of this region, the principal axis are extracted and assigned to instrument axis and instrument diameter. The diameter is used for depth approximation, i.e. distance of instrument tip to endoscope. The instrument pose is refined by initializing a 3D projection of the instrument with the extracted information and optimizing the overlap between projected model and image data by gradient descent. The described implementation requires more than 4.5 seconds per image. On a 97 frame in vivo dataset the overlap of the projected 3D model with a manual segmentation has an average precision[2] of 73.9%, a recall[3] of 67.1% and a probability of error[4] of 1.7%.

Loukas et al. (2013) [264] combine color marker tracking and instrument shaft tracking. Since only markerless approaches are discussed here, the former will not be discussed. The instrument shaft is tracked by a combination of straight line detection by Hough transform and a Kalman filter for tracking. The Kalman filter tracks the peaks corresponding to the most prominent straight lines, assumed to be the instrument shaft, in Hough space. This allows decrease the computational demands by only searching in a variance-defined vicinity $(2 \cdot \sigma)$ of the predicted shaft position. Results can not be compared to the other results in this section due to fusion with color marking tracking.

---

[2]Precision $= \frac{TP}{TP+FP}$ with the number of true positive (TP) and false positive (FP) classifications.

[3]Recall $= \frac{TP}{TP+FN}$ with the number of true positive (TP) and false negative (FN) classifications.

[4]Probability of error $PE = (TP + FN) \cdot FN + (TN + FP) \cdot FP$

Chen et al. (2013) [265] employ a spiking neural network with texture and geometric features for instrument detection and combine it with a Kalman filter. Edge features are detected by Laplacian of Gaussian (LoG) operator[5] a Gabor kernel is used to describe texture by frequency and orientation. The Kalman filter is used to narrow search in the image down by searching only in vicinity of the position predicted from the previous frame. Recognition rate on a 897 frames sequence is reported to be 91.9% and 99.1% for the right respective left instrument. Spatial accuracy is not reported.

Dockter et al. (2014) [266] perform 3D instrument tracking with stereo endoscopes. The probabilistic Hough transform is used to extract straight line segments from Sobel filtered images. Each pair of these is filtered according to a set of geometric condition thresholds (parallel, endpoint distance, distance to previous instrument position). The extracted instrument tips in the left and right camera are then used for a 3D reconstruction based on image disparity. Average in vivo tracking accuracy is 8.68 millimeters in 3D and 1.88 mm in 2D on a 54 second video clip. At least one tool was correctly detected 88% of the time and both tools 51.2% of the time.

Bodenstedt et al. [267] employ GPU-based random forests for pixel classification based on color features from multiple color spaces. Contours are extracted from the classified image. If two contours have a distance below a threshold they are fused into a larger one. The two largest contours if above a threshold are considered instruments. The furthest point from the contour center not on the image edge is selected as tip position. In case a stereo laparoscope is used, the tip points can be reconstructed from image disparity. Since the method is presented as part of a larger system, no results on instrument detection accuracy are provided.

All approaches described above are summarized in table 5.1. The implementation by Bodenstedt et al. has been integrated into the

---

[5]The combination of Gaussian smoothing and Laplacian filter for spatial derivation (edge enhancement).

modular platform (chapter 4) and has been utilized for training the knowledge-based camera guidance system presented here.

Table 5.1: Summary of approaches to markerless instrument tracking.

Year	Authors	Method	Reported results	Ref.
1994	Uecker et al.	Bayesian pixel classification; Connected regions; Simple shape analysis; Prediction next position; Tracking	Four $\leq$ 30 frame sequences: Error < 5% image size	[178]
2004	Climent et al.	Straight lines by Hough transform; Heuristic filter; Selection by metric on predicted position	128 frame sequence: 99% correct detection	[257]
2005	Doignon et al.	Color purity pixel classification; Sigma filter noise removal; Region growing; Closed contour Fourier descriptor region classification; Moments	—	[258]
2005	Kim et al.	Two-stage CONDENSATION tracking with modified adaptive color model	—	[259]

2006	Speidel et al.	Bayesian pixel classification; CONDENSATION tracking	100 frames: Error 82% 0.7% image size and 93% 1.4%	[260], [261]
2006	Voros et al.	Measurement of instrument trocar and projection into image plane; Straight lines to point by Hough transform	< 100 frame sequence: Error 70% < 2.5% image size and 80% < 5.5%	[202], [203]
2011	Wolf et al.	See Voros et al. 2006; CONDENSATION tracking	1050 frame sequence: Mean error 3.6% image size	[262]
2013	Allan et al.	Random forest pixel classification; Connected regions; Moments analysis; Optimization of 3D model projection	97 frame sequence: Precision 73.9%, recall 67.1%, probability of error 1.7%	[263]
2013	Loukas et al.	Shaft tracking: Straight lines by Hough transform; Kalman tracking in Hough space	Not comparable since fused with color marker tracking	[264]

2013	Chen et al.	Spiking neural network instrument recognition; Kalman tracking with search space reduction	897 frame sequence: Instrument recognition 91.9% and 99.1%	[265]
2014	Dockter et al.	Probabilistic Hough transform; Geometric condition thresholds on line pairs; Disparity 3D reconstruction	54 second video: Average error 3D 8.68 mm and 2D 1.88 mm; Correct detection of both tips 51.2% of at least one 88.0%	[266]
2015	Bodenstedt et al.	GPU-based random forest pixel classification; Contours extraction; Most distal point of largest contour	–	[267]

CVVisual

To improve the development process of computer vision applications, such as instrument tracking, I developed the CVVisual framework together with a number of undergraduate students. Only a brief synopsis is provided here, for more details see my paper [268] and the publicly available documentation[6]. CVVisual builds on the popular OpenCV framework[7] and provides *visual debugging* aids. Furthermore, it improves software engineering as ad-hoc debug code is replaced by short calls to the CVVisual API that do not require conditional preprocessor compilation in the application code for release mode (Fig. 5.3).

Ad-hoc debug code:
```
#ifdef DEBUG
  Mat img_matches;
  drawMatches(img1, keypoints1, img2, keypoints2,
              good_matches, img_matches, Scalar::all(-1),
              Scalar::all(-1), vector<char>(),
              DrawMatchesFlags::NOT_DRAW_SINGLE_POINTS);
  imshow("good matches", img_matches);
#endif
```

CVVisual replacement:
```
cvv:debugMatches(img1, img2, keypoints1, keypoints2, good_matches);
```

Figure 5.3: Example of how custom ad-hoc debug code, which is usually much longer in practice, can be replaced by calls to CV-Visual. While the former displays a static image, the later features an interactive multi-perspective GUI (Fig. 5.4).

When the first CVVisual debug call is encountered in the program, an overview GUI window is opened (Fig. 5.4a). Program flow is paused while the GUI is in use. The GUI allows to continue the program flow until the next debug call or run the program without interruption until a special finalizing call is encountered. A powerful engine for filtering and grouping the debug data is integrated into the overview window. Images can be viewed and zoomed down to the pixel level at which individual pixel values are overlaid. The important novel feature that facilitates iterative development is a set

---

[6]http://docs.opencv.org/trunk/. CVVisual is part of the official opencv_contrib repository.

[7]http://opencv.org

of complementary views each with multiple perspectives, which are available for inspection of related images.

The filter view (Fig. 5.4b) provides different perspectives on the result of a filter operation. For example, if a morphological transformation is applied to an image, the resulting images can be shown in an overlay, changed-pixel or difference perspective. In case of matches, which are calculated between two images, the match view (Fig. 5.4c) enables interactive exploration of the results. The figure shows parts of two laparoscopic images in which the endoscope was moved left. Although there are several wrong matches, the majority of matches between the instrument are quite good. The lines drawn are not static, but automatically adjust to zoom and pan in order to show the matches between the currently visible image parts. If the mouse is hovered over one of these match visualizations, additional information is provided.

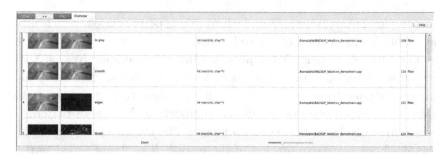

(a) Overview window of all debug calls.

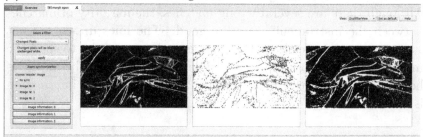

(b) Interactive filter view in dual perspective showing changed pixels.

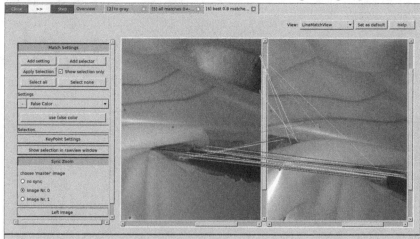

(c) Interactive match view in line perspective.

Figure 5.4: Screenshots from the CVVisual debug GUI.

5.2.2 Online Phase Recognition

A large amount of literature is available on (online) workflow analysis and (online) phase recognition of the surgical phase. These will not be surveyed here. Only a few recent approaches that are closely related to the implementation utilized in the endoscope guidance system are briefly described.

Speidel et al. (2008) [261] start with the extraction of information from endoscopic images, e.g. instrument trajectories and based on these activities. Description Logics (DL), in particular the web ontology language (OWL), are used to semantically describe the scene by means of the detected facts. The extracted information instantiates vocabulary from the terminology box (TBox) to populate the assertional box (ABox).[8] A DL reasoner matches the current ABox against situation descriptions in the TBox. The publication by Sudra et al. (2009) [270] extends the system by case-based reasoning (CBR). In CBR a similarity metric is defined on (symbolic) scene descriptions in order to match labeled cases to the current situation. Katic et al. [271] describe an extension of the system and apply it to dental surgery. Numeric measurements, for instance the distance between instrument and an anatomical structure, are mapped to symbolic values by learned fuzzy sets.

Weede et al. (2012) [272] combine information from tracked instruments, endoscope images and coagulation signal for online recognition of the surgical phase. A bag-of-words model (BoW) based on SIFT features is trained to recognize, but not localize, different instruments in the endoscopic image. Based on a nine phase workflow model of sigma resection, the occurrence and characteristics of certain features are learned for each phase. Features include instruments in use, statistics about their trajectories, coagulation characteristics as well as anatomical regions and time spent in the current phase. A set of Bayesian classifiers is trained that are indexed by the time spent in a phase, which can be seen as a Markov model with time-dependent

---

[8]See [269] for a detailed explanation of these terms.

transition probabilities. On a set of six interventions the true positive rate of phase detection compared to expert annotations is 93.2%.

5.3 Learning a Camera Guidance Quality Classifier

Learning a model of camera guidance know-how is posed as a problem of supervised learning: The input to the algorithm is a tuple (S, L) with S being being the set of samples $\{s_1, \ldots, s_N\}$ together with a corresponding set of labels $L = \{l_1, \ldots, l_N\}$. Each sample s_i consists of a feature vector $\mathbf{f}_j = (f_{j,1}, \ldots, f_{j,M})$. Labels are drawn from a finite discrete set of classes $\mathcal{C}$, i.e. $l_i \in L \subset \mathcal{C}$. The machine learning (ML) algorithm relates the samples S with the labels L in such a way that ideally for a sample s_i, which is not part of the training set $s_i \notin S$, the correct label l_i is predicted. One of the main challenges is to define a proper feature vector for spatial relations.

5.3.1 Learning Spatial Relations: A Static 1D Example

Before proceeding with a model for camera guidance, a simple one-dimensional example is provided here. The static spatial relation concerns three scalar points a, b and c. The point a is always left of point b. The relation to be learned is that c is supposed to be between a and b. If c is in between them and has a distance of at least δ to each, the position is assigned the label "good". If c is between a and b, but closer to either one, the position is labeled as "neutral". Otherwise the position is considered "poor". See Fig. 5.5 for an illustration of this spatial relation.

The most straight forward complete feature vector was chosen to represent the problem. Each sample is directly described by a tuple

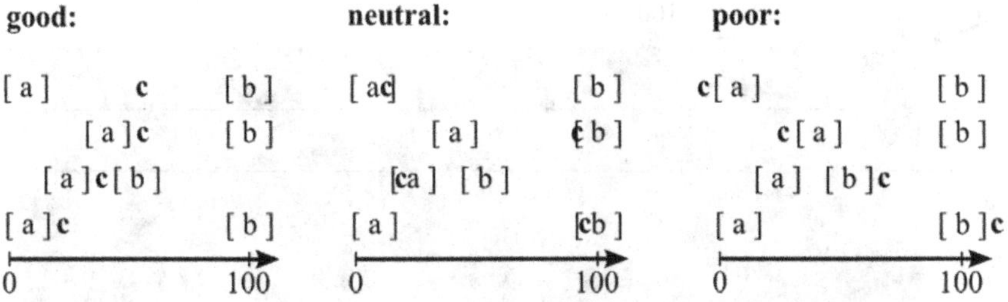

good: **neutral:**   **poor:**

[a]   c   [b]   [aᴄ]   [b]   c[a]   [b]

 [a]c   [b]   [a]   ₵b]   c[a]   [b]

 [a]c[b]   [ᴄa] [b]   [a] [b]c

[a]c   [b]   [a]   [ᴄb]   [a]   [b]c

0   100   0   100   0   100

Figure 5.5: Illustration of a simple static spatial relation to be learned: c is supposed to be between a and b with at least a distance of δ to both of them.

of the scalar values for each point $\mathbf{f} = (a, b, c)$. For the training set the labels are given by

$$l_i = \begin{cases} \text{good} & a + \delta < c < b - \delta \\ \text{neutral} & a < c \le a + \delta \vee b - \delta \le c < b \\ \text{poor} & \text{otherwise} \end{cases}$$

with $b - a > 2 * \delta$ and $\delta = 5$. The generated training set did not contain any mislabeled items. My ClassIt framework for optimization of meta-parameters in machine learning algorithms was used for training (see 5.3.4).[9] The results are shown in Fig. 5.6.

The rightmost result for 100.000 training samples is very close to the ground truth. Looked at the other way round, the simple problem for a training set that does not contain noise or mislabeled items, already requires 100.000 training instances in order to capture the spatial relation properly. Repeating the same experiment, but this time with a slightly modified feature vector $\mathbf{f} = (a, b, c, a - c, b - c)$, results for smaller training data sets are improved (Fig. 5.7). Yet, still about 10.000 samples are required. Finally, if the feature vector is extended by a field that nearly captures the spatial criteria in a logical formula by itself, $\mathbf{f} = (a, b, c, a - c, b - c, (a < c) \wedge (c < b))$, acceptable results can be achieved with around 1.000 samples.

---

[9]Settings used: Classifiers = {Random Forests}; maxDepth = 3:[10,20]; maxTrees 5:[10,100]; trainTestRatio=0.9

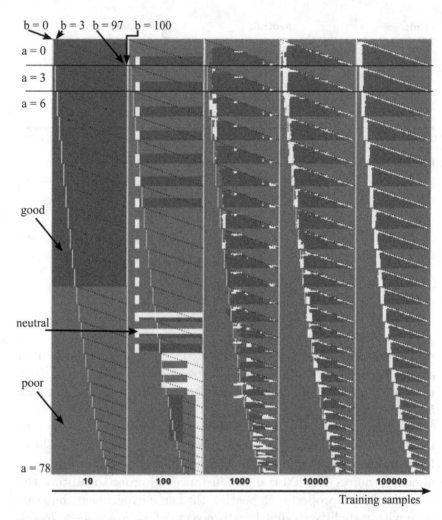

Figure 5.6: Results for learning a static, one-dimensional spatial relationship with different training set sizes. Feature vector
$\mathbf{f} = (a, b, c)$. Point a is shown as a white pixel □, b is shown
as black pixel ■. The predicted label for c is shown by pixel
color: good, neutral and poor.

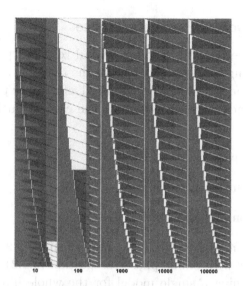

Figure 5.7: See Fig. 5.6, here the results for feature vector $\mathbf{f} = (a, b, c, a - c, b - c)$ are shown.

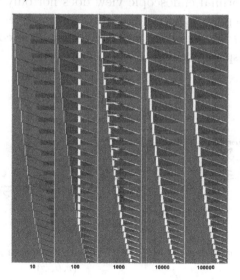

Figure 5.8: See Fig. 5.6, here the results for feature vector $\mathbf{f} = (a, b, c, a - c, b - c, (a < c) \wedge (c < b))$ are shown.

5.3.2 Reduction of Parameter Space

As shown in the previous section, spatial relations pose a complex
machine learning problem. Therefore, the dynamic spatial relation
that is to be modeled should be simplified as much as possible. Three
different methods were employed for the camera quality classifiers
(CQC):

- Step-specific models

- Projective dimension reduction

- Normalization and binarization by thresholding

Step-specific models are feasible due to using a surgical workflow
(3.2.3) together with online phase recognition (5.2.2) in the system.
Instead of learning a single model for the whole intervention, one
model per surgical step is learned. The relation between instrument
position and optimal endoscopic view does not only change within
each surgical step (short-term), but also between different steps (long-
term). Thus the ML algorithm must only learn a less complex relation
in case of step specific models.

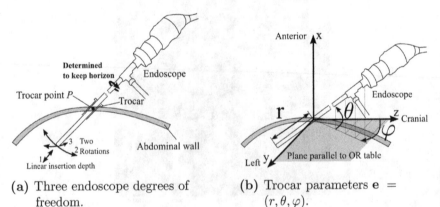

(a) Three endoscope degrees of freedom.

(b) Trocar parameters $\mathbf{e} = (r, \theta, \varphi)$.

Figure 5.9: Representation of endoscope positions.

A rigid object without symmetries has six degrees of freedom in positioning. Due to the trocar constraint (cf. Fig. 1.10) an endoscope has only four degrees of freedom while inserted into the trocar. However, by utilizing factual (textbook) knowledge about endoscope guidance (cf. 3.2.3) one further degree of freedom can be eliminated by projection and later on unambiguously recovered (Fig. 5.9a).[10] Overall, the endoscope parameters $\mathbf{e}$ can be described by three scalars $\mathbf{e} = (r, \theta, \varphi)$ (Fig. 5.9b).

Given the endoscope pose P in homogeneous coordinates and the translational position of the camera trocar $\mathbf{t}$ in a common coordinate system, the endoscope parameters are given by Eq. 5.1[11]:

$$\mathbf{d} = \mathbf{t} - P[1, 3; 4]$$
$$r = \|\mathbf{d}\|$$
$$\theta = \arccos(\frac{\mathbf{d}_z}{r}) \qquad (5.1)$$
$$\phi = \arctan(\frac{\mathbf{d}_y}{\mathbf{d}_x})$$

The inverse direction, from endoscope parameters $\mathbf{e}$ to a 6D endoscope pose P as a homogeneous matrix is given by Eq. 5.2,5.3:

$$\mathbf{p} = \begin{pmatrix} r \cdot \sin(\theta) \cdot \cos(\phi) \\ r \cdot \sin(\theta) \cdot \sin(\phi) \\ r \cdot \cos(\theta) \end{pmatrix}$$
$$\mathbf{u} = (-1, 0, 0)^\mathsf{T} \qquad (5.2)$$
$$\mathbf{z} = \frac{\mathbf{p}}{\|\mathbf{p}\|}$$
$$\mathbf{x} = \frac{\mathbf{u} \times \mathbf{z}}{\|\mathbf{u} \times \mathbf{z}\|}$$

---

[10]It is assumed that 0° optics are used.

[11]The notation $M[a, b; c, d]$ allows to specify submatrices, it denotes the matrix given as the intersection of rows $\{a, \ldots, b\}$ and columns $\{c, \ldots, d\}$.

$$\mathbf{y} = \frac{\mathbf{z} \times \mathbf{x}}{\|\mathbf{z} \times \mathbf{x}\|}$$

$$P = \begin{pmatrix} \mathbf{x}, & \mathbf{y}, & \mathbf{z}, & \mathbf{p}+\mathbf{t} \\ 0, & 0, & 0, & 1 \end{pmatrix} \tag{5.3}$$

The rotation along the endoscope shaft is determined in order to keep the camera horizon parallel to the global coordinate system, e.g. the OR floor or OR table.

At this point, three elements of the feature vector are given by (r, θ, φ) and encode all required information about the endoscope position. The other information to be encoded are the instrument positions. Experimental evaluation of different encodings resulted in the chosen feature vector shown in Eq. 5.4:

$$\mathbf{f} = \left(\underbrace{r, \theta, \varphi,}_{e} \underbrace{n}_{\text{No. exist}}, \underbrace{e_1, v_1, \hat{x}_1, \hat{y}_1,}_{\text{1st instrument}} \underbrace{e_2, v_2, \hat{x}_2, \hat{y}_2,}_{\text{2nd instrument}} \underbrace{e_3, v_3, \hat{x}_3, \hat{y}_3}_{\text{3rd instrument}} \right) \tag{5.4}$$

The number n is an integer that counts the number of instruments currently in use. Each instrument is encoded by 4 values $(e_i, v_i, \hat{x}_i, \hat{y}_i)$ in the feature vector. e_i is an categorical boolean variable and encodes whether the instrument is currently in use. Thus, $n = \sum_i e_i$. The value v_i is also a categorical boolean variable and encodes whether the instrument tip is visible, i.e. within the endoscope's field of view. Finally, $(\hat{x}_i, \hat{y}_i)$ are the image position of the visible instruments normalized to $[-0.5, 0.5]$ around the image center from image resolution $w \times h$ dependent pixel position (x_i, y_i) (Eq. 5.5):

$$(\hat{x}_i, \hat{y}_i) = \begin{cases} \left(\frac{x_i - w/2}{w}, \frac{y_i - h/2}{h} \right) & x_i \leq w \wedge y_i \leq h \\ (\infty, \infty) & \text{otherwise} \end{cases} \tag{5.5}$$

5.3.3 Deriving Synthetic Learning Examples

Having described the feature vector of the camera quality classifier (CQC), the next topic to discuss is class imbalance in the training data. The problem with datasets in minimally-invasive surgery is that they cannot be performed under an highly unsuited endoscopic view just to train a classifier. The challenges of camera guidance (cf. 1.1.2) often result in suboptimal endoscopic views during the intervention. Yet, these do not occur to the same extent as good or at least neutral endoscope positions. Furthermore, there are no examples of very poor endoscope positioning in the training data, such as the endoscope pointing in the opposite direction of the instruments. Still these examples, which represent endoscope positions that are obviously wrong for a human camera assistant, help the machine learning algorithm to make better predictions, especially in regions of the feature space that are only sparely explored by training samples.

In Fig. 5.10 training data from a single intervention was used to train a camera quality classifier. In the upper image (Fig. 5.10a) the CQC was trained without synthetic samples. Since many areas of the feature space are not covered at all by the training data, prediction in these areas is effectively random. Thus even endoscope positions that face away from the instruments can be classified as suitable. In contrast the lower image (Fig. 5.10b) shows the sampling of a CQC trained on the same recorded data, but this time with additional synthetic data that is generated from the recorded one. Here all endoscope positions classified as good are at least plausible candidates.

For generation of synthetic learning samples, factual knowledge was combined with a geometric consideration. For each sample in the recorded intervention data that was annotated as a good endoscope position by the surgeon, synthetic samples are generated in the following manner: The instrument tips are transfered in a parent coordinate frame of the endoscope, e.g. the external tracker or the fixed trocar coordinate system. Starting with a manually specified threshold t_a, an offset grid with step size δ_a is applied to the endoscope parameters **e** (see 5.3.2 above) while keeping the instrument position fixed with

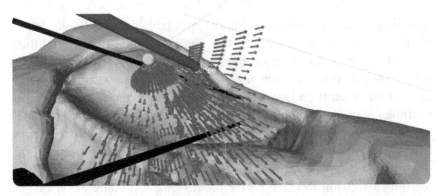

(a) No use of synthetic learning samples: Unexplored areas of the feature space are often considered "good" positions.

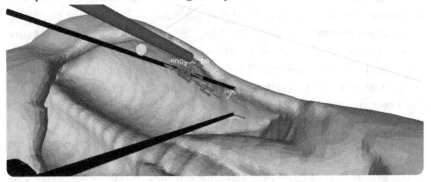

(b) With synthetic learning samples: No unexplored areas in feature space.

Figure 5.10: Illustration how synthetic learning samples improve machine learning performance for camera quality classifiers.

respect to the parent coordinate system (Eq. 5.6).

$$
\begin{aligned}
\{\mathbf{e}' = (r', \theta', \varphi') \, | & \, r' = \delta_r \cdot i, 0.01 \leq r' \leq 0.35, |r - r'| > t_r, \\
& \theta' = \delta_\theta \cdot i, \frac{\pi}{2} \leq \theta' \leq \pi, |\theta - \theta'| > t_\theta, \\
& \varphi' = \delta_\varphi \cdot i, -\pi \leq \varphi' \leq \pi, |\varphi - \varphi'| > t_\varphi, \\
& i \in \mathbb{Z}\}
\end{aligned}
\tag{5.6}
$$

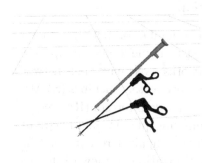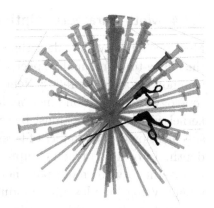

(a) Relation of endoscope and instruments in training data labeled as "good".

(b) Illustration of synthetic "poor" training data generated from recorded data.

Figure 5.11: Visualization of synthetic endoscope positions for synthetic training samples. Note: The actual grid step size δ_a is much smaller, i.e. much more synthetic positions are generated (shown: 100; actual: 2400).

Instruments positions in the endoscope image, i.e. the instrument features in **f**, are recomputed based on the modified **e**. The resulting transformation is a virtual repositioning of the endoscope for the recorded instrument positions (Fig. 5.11). Thresholds are chosen sufficiently large to render it very likely that the synthetic endoscope position can be assigned the label "poor". Because there are many more ways to position the endoscope wrong than there are good positions or at least plausible candidate positions, after the above process, there are much more synthetic samples than recorded data. However, this does not pose a problem since all synthetic positions are directly derived from actual data. Furthermore, most of the synthetic data resides in parts of the feature space that do not contain any recorded data.

5.3.4 Meta-Parameter Optimization

Most machine learning algorithms have a number of meta-parameters that have to be manually specified. Just to name a few examples for common algorithm families: Neural networks (NN) have their network topology and activation function; for support vector machines (SVM) a kernel with parameters must be selected; random forests (RF) require specification of the number of trees, minimum split size and maximum depth. In order to trade computation time against researcher time, a straight forward meta-parameter optimization framework for the OpenCV machine learning module was developed. This framework, named ClassIt, provides a uniform API to several machine learning algorithms such as the ones mentioned above. Furthermore, the range of each meta-parameters for each algorithm to be evaluated can be specified. After passing all training samples and labels to ClassIt, all combinations of algorithms and meta-parameters are evaluated in parallel[12]. Evaluation of classifier performance is done by splitting the user-provided data into a training and a test set with a user-defined ratio. The best classifier, that is combination of ML algorithm and meta-parameters, is returned. Many classifiers also have a tradeoff between classification quality and performance. For example, the classification runtime for random forests is linear in the number of trees and in their depth. ClassIt also allows to pick other classifiers given a multi-objective criterion, like a classifier from the runtime-quality Pareto frontier.

Random forests [273] turned out to be superior for learning spatial relations in terms of a camera quality classifier (CQC). Therefore, only their meta-parameters were optimized in later iterations. Optimal parameters for the training data sets used in the evaluation (see chapter 7) were found to be about 50 trees with a maximum depth of 20. As can be seen from table 5.2, the absolute prediction error varies with the surgical step for which a CQC is trained.

---

[12]Currently only shared-memory parallelism is implemented, i.e. all processors on a single machine are utilized, but computation is not distributed across multiple machines.

Table 5.2: The table shows the average percentage prediction error for a 3-fold repeated random sub-sampling validation for three surgical steps from the evaluation data (chapter 7). Train to test split ratio is set to 90%. The number of samples for the steps are 1.056.283 for colon, 1.205.875 for artery and 1.424.658 for dissect rectum. Data sets included synthetic samples as described in 5.3.3. All numbers given as percentage and rounded to two decimal places.

Step	Tree depth	Number of Trees				
		10	32	55	77	100
Colon	10	0.72	0.64	0.59	0.60	0.62
	15	0.37	0.37	0.36	0.35	0.36
	20	0.50	0.35	0.32	0.31	0.30
Artery	10	1.14	1.15	1.16	1.12	1.13
	15	0.99	0.90	0.91	0.93	0.91
	20	0.95	0.87	0.86	0.86	0.86
Dissect Rectum	10	1.29	1.26	1.21	1.21	1.21
	15	1.05	0.99	0.98	0.97	0.97
	20	0.98	0.87	0.87	0.87	0.86

5.3.5 Classifier Evaluation: Point in Time and Period of Time

As described above, the camera quality classifier (CQC) was trained with respect to predictive error on the training dataset. That is, for each point in time, the relation between endoscope and surgical instruments is matched to the expert labels. However, it is not clear whether a classifier with the lowest predictive error is also the best one for intraoperative camera guidance. The reason is that while the former is an instantaneous perspective, camera guidance is performed over a period of time. Intraoperatively, the CQC is continuously sampled and the results influence the following queries (see the following chapter).

In contrast to for example image classification, performance evaluation on a static benchmark set, i.e. only measuring the instantaneous prediction error, is unlikely to capture camera guidance performance. Instead I propose to run the full intraoperative algorithm against a benchmark dataset, record the resulting virtual endoscopic view and have the video labeled by experts in the same manner as the training data was created.

6 Intraoperative Robot-Based Camera Assistance

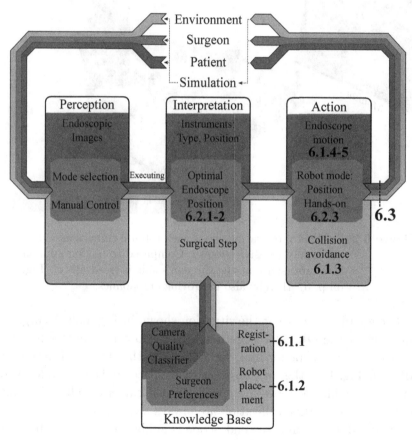

Figure 6.1: Overview of chapter 6 (cf. Fig. 3.7 p. 113).

In this chapter the two remaining components required for an intraoperative camera assistance are discussed: First, the necessary preliminaries to utilize the modular platform that was discussed in chapter 4 for endoscope positioning (6.1). Second, how the learned camera guidance model is deployed for optimal endoscope positioning over time (6.2).

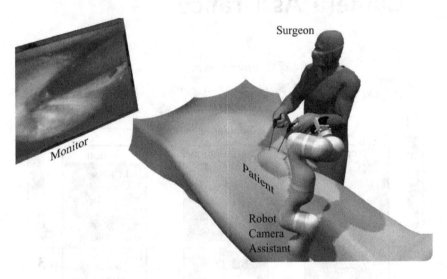

Figure 6.2: Outline of operating room with robotic camera assistance in minimally-invasive surgery. Compared to having a human assistant, space at the surgeon's side is freed up (cf. Fig. 1.1 on p. 3), thereby also improving ergonomics.

The goal is to arrive at the situation shown in Fig. 6.2: A surgeon operates at the OR table together with a robot that autonomously guides the endoscope for him. In contrast to the current situation in MIS (cf. Fig. 1.1), the surgeon gains more space at the OR table. The endoscope guidance know-how encoded in the camera quality classifier and its intraoperative utilization are always at the same performance level. In addition, once the endoscope is guided by a robot, optional action components are available (6.3), such as dynamically extending the field of view.

Figure 6.1 shows the structure of this chapter with respect to the overall camera guidance system.

6.1 Preliminaries

6.1.1 Calibration and Registration

A number of standard calibration and registration problems have to be solved for robot-assisted camera guidance. The methods used are summarized here.

Endoscope Camera Calibration

The endoscope camera and optics are intrinsically calibrated (Fig. 6.3) with the standard ROS tool for camera_calibration[1] using a checkerboard calibration target. This tool is based on the OpenCV calibration module (calib3d), which in turn uses the algorithm by Zhang et al. [274]. Two variants have been implemented:

- Manual: The robot keeps the endoscope static and the calibration target is moved by hand in front of the endoscope until a sufficient set of different perspectives has been captured.

- Automatic: The calibration target is placed on the OR table and the robot automatically positions the endoscope in order to capture different perspectives.[2]

Hand-Eye Calibration

Hand-Eye calibration refers to calibrating the transformation from the robot coordinate system to the camera coordinate system (Fig. 6.4). After intrinsic calibration of the endoscope, this is a standard problem of robotics. Several options are available in ROS, of these

---

[1]http://wiki.ros.org/camera_calibration

[2]This assumes, at least an approximate, prior robot to endoscope (hand-eye) calibration.

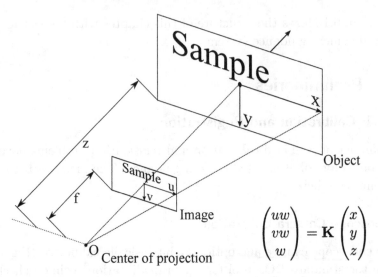

$$\begin{pmatrix} uw \\ vw \\ w \end{pmatrix} = \mathbf{K} \begin{pmatrix} x \\ y \\ z \end{pmatrix}$$

Figure 6.3: Illustration of the problem solved by intrinsic calibration: Projection of 3D world coordinates to 2D image coordinates by the camera matrix K. Typically, also parameters of a radial distortions model are fitted during calibration, which allow to undistort the image (not shown).

visp_hand2eye_calibration[3] package and furthermore the powerful industrial_extrinsic_cal[4] package have been evaluated. Apart from practical issues due to the long distance between robot flange and camera projection center, due of the long endoscope shaft, both packages solve the problem with sufficient accuracy. No further evaluation than visual inspection of the reprojection error was performed.

---

[3]http://wiki.ros.org/vision_visp using the ViSP framework (http://visp.inria.fr).

[4]http://wiki.ros.org/industrial_extrinsic_cal. The package can also solve different kinds of calibration problems by formulating them as a large nonlinear least squares problems (bundle adjustment) and solving them with Google's Ceres solver.

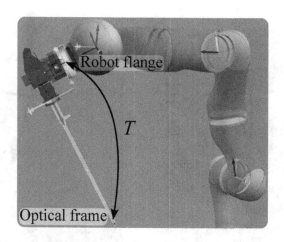

Figure 6.4: The hand-eye calibration problem: Calculating the transform T between the robot and camera coordinate system.

Robot to Trocar Registration

In the current system, it is assumed that the camera trocar is always placed in the umbilicus. Thus no registration of trocar to patient is required. If the camera trocar must to be freely placeable, any registration method that achieves an accuracy of a few centimeters can be used. No higher accuracy is required because all calculations in terms of endoscope to instruments relation occur relative to the trocar frame. As long as the same surgical tasks are performed in the same regions relative to the trocar, the camera quality classifier is sufficiently generic to work well.

In contrast, the robot to trocar registration must be performed with a much higher accuracy. Depending on whether the KUKA LWR or the ViKY is used for endoscope positioning, the trocar is registered to the robot in a different manner. In case of the ViKY, which is directly placed over the trocar (cf. Fig. 2.16a), the translational registration is already performed during placement of the robot. The rotational registration is performed by rotating the ViKY until the endoscope

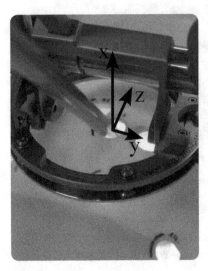
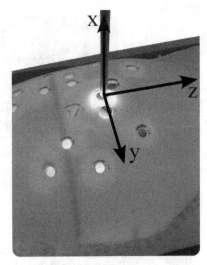

(a) ViKY: Translational registration is given by placement of
the robot, rotational one by
initial alignment to z-axis.

(b) LWR: Registration is performed by pointing the endoscope tip at the trocar point.
Rotation is given by rigid
attachment of robot to table.

Figure 6.5: Trocar registration procedure for ViKY and LWR.

faces straight along the z-axis[5] (Fig. 6.5a). The LWR is registered to
the trocar by moving the endoscope in hands-on mode into the trocar
and inserting it until the tip is at level of the abdominal wall. Since
the LWR is assumed to be mounted to the OR table rail, the rotation
with respect to the patient is sufficiently well known (Fig. 6.5b).
Alternatively, if the LWR can be freely placed with respect to the
patient, the same procedure as for the ViKY can be utilized.

6.1.2 Trocar and Robot Placement

The optimal placement of camera trocar and instrument trocars, in
terms of reachability, dexterity and ergonomics, is an active field of

---

[5]The z-axis faces cranial, cf. Fig. 1.7.

research in itself (cf. [275]). In case of robot-assisted MIS, another question is the placement of the robot relative to the trocars. The most important criterion is whether the robot can reach all positions that are relevant for a particular intervention.

For the ViKY the reachability question is easy to answer because its spherical kinematics (cf. 2.1.9) enable it, in principle, to reach any position within the trocar. In principle, because the endoscope or the structure holding it can collide with the instruments and is thus blocked from reaching certain positions.

Whether all position are reachable is not as easy to answer for a robot with different kinematics such as the LWR. Largely due to joint limits[6], not all poses in the robot's workspace are reachable. The number of unreachable poses on a specific path is even larger. In MIS the trocar constraint (cf. Fig. 1.10) must be adhered to at all times and usually a straight spherical motion is demanded as well. This often leads to dead ends of the intraoperative robot motion, which can be very frustrating for the OR staff since the kinematical limits are often not obvious.

Therefore, a preoperative optimization of the robot placement is investigated by Hutzl et al. [277][276]. An approach based on recorded intervention trajectories is pursued. Given a kinematical model of the robot together with the attached endoscope, the reachability of all positions in the recorded trajectories can be virtually assessed. This is used to find the optimal placement of the robot at the OR table relative to the trocar.

---

[6]For other robot kinematics another important reason are self-collisions.

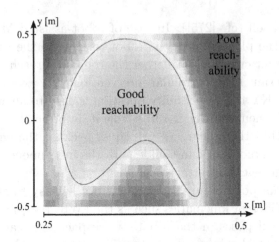

Figure 6.6: Reachability index for the LWR when positioning the robot in different places relative to the trocar (x-y plane) for a fixed height of the trocar (see [276]). Positions that lead to a good reachability are indicated together with those resulting in less reachable positions in the recorded intervention data.

6.1.3 Collision Avoidance

Basic collision avoidance is implemented using the MoveIt framework (cf. 4.1). This includes self collisions of the robot and to the known static environment, including the OR table. Furthermore, MoveIt allows to include point cloud streams, e.g. provided by time of flight or depth cameras, into the collision checking. This can be used to avoid collision of the robot with the OR staff. Because there are many occlusions around the OR table, a fixed multi camera setup mounted at the ceiling, as available in the modular platform (see 4.2.2), could be applied to this task. However, this was not a focus of the thesis at hand.

Another important type of collisions are collisions between the robot-guided endoscope and the patient's abdominal organs. Unfortunately, no solution that guarantees this under all circumstances is available. Therefore, three safety layers in the camera guidance system have been implemented that close this gap as good as possible until a future solution becomes available:

- The maximum robot velocity is limited in a ROS node independent of the camera guidance commands.

- The maximum extends of endoscope motion are learned from recorded intervention data for each surgical step and adhered to intraoperatively.

- The camera quality classifiers learn that in all good endoscope positions at least one instrument is in front of the endoscope tip.

A fourth safety layer that would provide additional safety could be implemented with a stereo endoscope. By calculating the minimum distance between tissue and endoscope tip from the disparity images, a reactive behavior could be added as additional action component (cf. 6.3) that always maintains a minimum distance.

6.1.4 Basic Robot Performance

Camera motion results in motion blur and should thus be avoided, unless the motion is required to change the field of view. One particular kind of motion that is never intentional is tremor in case of a human assistant and vibrations in case of robot assistance. I evaluated the latter with respect to the three robots that are integrated into the modular platform (cf. Fig. 3.14) and used for autonomous endoscope guidance [278].

Given a simple pinhole camera model, such as the one shown in Fig. 6.3, an order of magnitude estimate for endoscope cameras looks as follows: A length L in meters (m) on the object plane, is mapped to a image length l in pixels (px) given by $l = \frac{f}{z} \cdot L$. For a 10mm laparoscope with low zoom, intrinsic calibration results in $f = 955$px. A common distance between endoscope tip and scene objects is on the order of $0.1m$. Thus $l \approx \frac{1000\text{px}}{0.1m} \cdot L$. If the camera motion during exposure time is less than one pixel, no visible motion blur occurs. Given an estimated exposure time of $t_e = 0.01s$, the maximum velocity

v_{max} at which no motion blur occurs, assuming a simple translational motion, is given by $v_{max} = \frac{L_{max}}{t_e} = \frac{0.0001m}{0.01s} = 0.01\frac{m}{s}$.

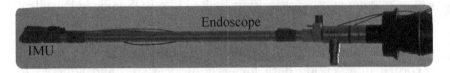

Figure 6.7: Vibration measurement setup: A small IMU (1 g) attached to the endoscope tip.

A small inertial measurement unit (IMU), weighting about 1 g, was attached to the distal endoscope end (Fig. 6.7). Given a sampling rate of the accelerometer contained in the IMU of 570 Hz, a lower bound for the high frequency instantaneous velocities of the endoscope tip due to vibration is given as $\tilde{v} = 9.81\frac{m}{s^2} \cdot \frac{1}{570}$Hz $\cdot a$ with a being the measured acceleration.

The raw acceleration data (Fig. 6.8a) was first modified to have a zero mean by subtracting the sliding window average (Fig. 6.8b) Afterwards a histogram of this data was computed (Fig. 6.8c).

Measurements were taken for different trocar compliant robot motions (Fig. 6.9). To simulate the dampening influence of the trocar, some motions were performed through a silicone trocar in a medical phantom. Overall it was found that no robot causes motion blur due to vibrations most of time when inserted into a trocar. Even then the largest detected blur was on the order of 2 pixels, which is only visible on the monitor under ideal viewing conditions.

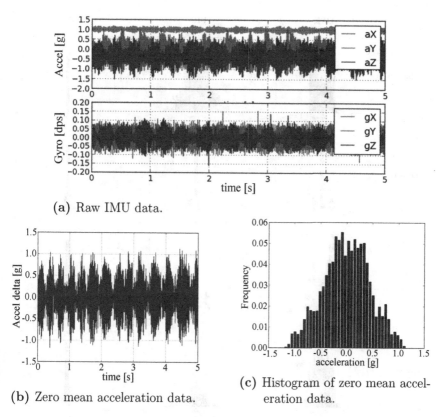

(a) Raw IMU data.

(b) Zero mean acceleration data.

(c) Histogram of zero mean acceleration data.

Figure 6.8: Processing from raw IMU data to vibration histograms.

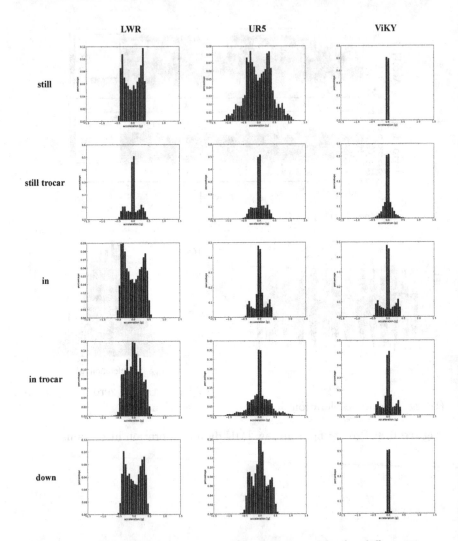

Figure 6.9: Vibration histograms of the endoscope tip for different motions of the robots in the modular platform. Note that not the robots are assessed by themselves, but the combination of robot and endoscope attachment and in case of motions also the control.

6.1.5 Mapping to Spherical Coordinates

For the LWR and the UR5 a mapping to spherical coordinates and trocar compliant motion is required. In order to have unified interfaces to these robots and the ViKY, a custom message type was defined that uses the trocar parameter representation **e** (cf. 5.3.2). In case of the other robots a separate node maps the trocar parameters to Cartesian coordinates using their unified ROS interface (cf. 4.7 and Fig. 6.10). This node also performs interpolation in spherical coordinates.

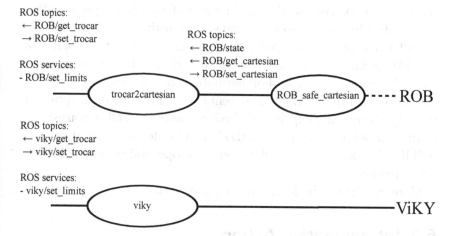

Figure 6.10: Unified ROS interface for endoscope positioning using the LWR, UR5 and ViKY. ROB is a variable for {lwr,ur5}.

6.1.6 Modeling and Execution of Surgical Workflow

Based on my earlier work on planning with hierarchical task networks (HTNs) [279], I propose to use HTNs as a novel workflow modeling language.

A task network $w = (U, C)$ consists of a task set U with precedence, before, between and after constraints C. An HTN method $m =$ (name, task, subtasks, constraints) is applied to w by decomposing a task into subtasks and extending C by constraints. A planning problem

$P = (s_0, w, O, M)$ starts in the initial state s_0. Operators O and methods M are used to compute a plan π, which contains an ordered set of ground primitive tasks, whose execution does not violate any constraints.

The approach unifies workflow modeling and planning by basing the surgical workflow modeling domain-specific language (DSL) on HTNs. Thus, the HTN planner can automatically check the modeled workflow for consistency and operability. This HTN-based DSL has three important properties: First, it is inherently hierarchical, easing modeling of complex workflows in contrast to a flat representation. Second, it is local and reusable because its constituents are defined in a modular manner without global dependencies. Third, the description provides an implicit representation of all workflows that are compatible with the domain model. Furthermore, existing ontologies can be transformed into the HTN representation. The planning approach provides the domain expert with feedback about workflow consistency during modeling. Abstract methods can be defined and utilized as building blocks, while the planer ensures operability on the level of primitive tasks.

More details can be found in my paper [280].

6.2 Intraoperative Action

This section describes how the camera quality classifier (CQC), which has been learned in chapter 5, is utilized intraoperatively to guide the endoscope. The outer functions of the algorithm are summarized as pseudocode in Fig. 6.11.

```
01:   def guidance_loop():   // 6.2.2
02:     while running:
03:       pose, endoscope, instrument = currentScene()
04:       features = describe(endoscope, instruments)
05:       best_local = bestLocalPose(features)
06:       best_global = bestGlobalPose(features)
07:       best_pose = combine(best_local, best_global, w_lg)
08:       next_pose = combine(best_pose, pose, w_speed)
09:       if memory.distance(next_pose) > τ_m:
10:         memory.add(next_pose)
11:         move(next_pose)
12:       memory.update(timestep)
13:
14:   def bestLocalPose(features):   // 6.2.1
15:     Δ = (δ_r, δ_θ, δ_φ) = sampler.range(last_good_count)
16:     e = features.endoscope
18:     return bestPose(features, (e - Δ, e + Δ))
19:
20:   def bestPose(features, range):
21:     predictions = predictGrid(features, range)
22:     good_poses = extractGood(predictions)
23:     return average(good_poses)
24:
25:   def predictGrid(features, range):   // 5.3.2
26:     r⁻, r⁺ = range
27:     return { (e',q) | r⁻ ≤ e' ≤ r⁺,
28:       q = cqc.predict(features.update(e')) }
```

Figure 6.11: Pseudocode of how the next best endoscope position is computed in the knowledge-based camera guidance. In the implementation several of these steps run in parallel using a producer-consumer scheme.

6.2.1 Inverting the Forward Model by Adaptive Sampling

As described in section 5.3, the camera quality classifier (CQC) maps from features $\mathbf{f}$, describing the endoscope position $\mathbf{e}$ and instrument positions, to a quality $q \in \{\text{good}, \text{neutral}, \text{bad}\}$. Yet, the intraoperative goal is to go from a given $\mathbf{f}$ to an optimal endoscope position $\mathbf{e}^*$. This is achieved by sampling different endoscope positions $\mathbf{e}'$ and computing a new feature vector $\mathbf{f}'$ for them. The sampling can be seen as virtually moving the endoscope while keeping the instrument in the same absolute position. The number of samples $|s|$ is a multiplicative function of the spatial coverage Δ and the sampling density ρ: $|s| = \Delta \cdot \rho$. Given a fixed amount of computational power, e.g. all cores of a modern desktop computer for one 10th of a second, the number of samples that can be evaluated is fixed $|s| = \text{const}$. The result is that either the sampling coverage or the sampling density can be increased while the other must be decreased at the same time.

Thus, adaptive sampling, using a fixed number of samples, is applied to the CQC. Starting with an initial coverage Δ_0, the coverage is adjusted (and correspondingly the density in the other way) for each query in the following manner:

$$\Delta_{t+1} = \begin{cases} \max(\Delta_{\min}, \Delta_t \cdot \sigma_-) & |q_g| > \tau_+ \\ \min(\Delta_{\max}, \Delta_t \cdot \sigma_+) & |q_g| < \tau_- \\ \Delta_t & \text{otherwise} \end{cases}$$

with $|q_g|$ being the number of samples classified as good by the CQC, $\Delta_{\min}$ and $\Delta_{\max}$ as upper and lower coverage bound, σ_* as scaling factors and τ_* as upper and lower threshold. The result is that the optimal endoscope pose can be narrowed down to any precision utilizing only a fixed amount of computation time. If the optimal position is lost, the searched parameter space is automatically widened to regain an initial estimate. In Fig. 6.12 this process is visualized.

The candidate good endoscope positions for different surgical steps and thereby different learned CQCs are illustrated in Fig. 6.13.

In order to get out of local optima, an independent low-density sampling is performed with global coverage. These are combined after separate fusion of local candidate poses and global ones (see line 07 in Fig. 6.11).

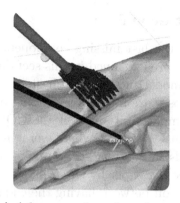 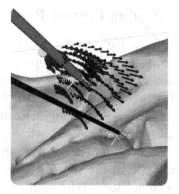

(a) A large number of good positions is predicted in the vicinity of the current endoscope position. The sampling coverage is decreased and the sampling density increased.

(b) If not enough positions are labeled as good by the CQC in the currently sampled space, the sampling coverage is increased, thereby decreasing the sampling density.

Figure 6.12: Visualization of the adaptive sampling process.

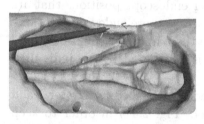 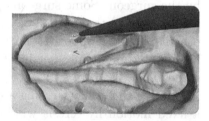

(a) Mobilization sigmoid.

(b) Mobilization splenic flexure.

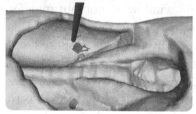 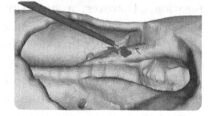

(c) Division of artery.

(d) Dissection of rectum.

Figure 6.13: Illustration of CQC sampling in different surgical steps.

6.2.2 From Current Pose to Next Good Pose

Referring back to Fig. 3.11 (p. 120), the last missing components for autonomous endoscope positioning are explained in this section: fusion of candidate positions, motion model and decaying hysteresis.

In the current system, candidate poses are fused by averaging of the endoscope parameters **e** of all sample positions that the CQC evaluates as good. However, care must be taken when averaging orientations as there are many pitfalls in contrast to averaging of translations. For more information, see the paper by Olsen [281]).

The motion model realizes the trade-off between having the endoscope in minimum distance to the optimal position and keeping a steady camera image. If being in the optimal position is considered more important, the endoscope must move more often and more quickly. In the other extreme, a perfectly stable camera never moves at all. The motion model allows to linearly interpolate between these two extremes by weighting the resulting position (see w_{speed} in Fig. 6.11). This parameter can also be made available for control by the surgeon. Some surgeons prefer endoscope positions that are always close to the optimal one and accept more endoscope motions, others prefer the opposite. Therefore the parameter could be stored in a profile preference setting that is associated to the individual surgeon.[7]

Many of the visual servoing approaches described in chapter 2 add a fixed motion hysteresis window (cf. Fig. 2.41) in order to keep the endoscope position static for small variations of the instrument position. However, a static hysteresis window is not optimal for the situationally adaptive endoscope positioning described in this thesis. Therefore, a time-decaying motion hysteresis is proposed and implemented in the system. A position memory stores the target position of every endoscope motion initiated by the system (see lines 09-12 in Fig. 6.11). If the next endoscope position is too close to a previously stored one, the endoscope is not moved. In each time

---

[7]Another such surgeon preferences that might be worth investigating for similar reasons is a proportional zoom offset.

step the oldest positions are removed. As an effect the endoscope can, in contrast to a fixed hysteresis window, remain in a suboptimal position only for a limited time period. In addition, the size of the position memory is bounded. The proposed approach can lead to limit cycles, however, these are very unlikely due to the dynamic nature of instrument motions and have a very low frequency in case they do occur.

6.2.3 Multimodal Human-Robot-Interaction

The interaction between the surgeon and the knowledge-based camera guidance can be broken up into control of mode and manual control of endoscope position. Multiple interfaces using different modalities were implemented because each interface is better suited for some tasks and less for others. This is best illustrated with an example: Fig. 6.14 shows how task-dependent the usability of a particular interface is. It is easy to command the system, e.g. by voice command, to center on the right instrument tip because only symbolic positions and actions are involved: "Center on right instrument". On the other hand, the second task indicated in the figure pertains to an anatomical structure that is not known by the system and thus has no label attached to it. Control by voice would involve quantitative spatial relations, e.g. "Move endoscope 1 cm to the left and 5.8 cm down". However, while it is easy for the system to exactly reposition the endoscope as commanded, it is very difficult for the surgeon to utilize such quantities[8]. Therefore, providing a multimodal interface to the surgeon allows to utilize the modality best suited to the particular task. In the above example, the second task could be easily accomplished by a continuous subsymbolic modality such as a foot pedal or a joystick. For an overview on user interfaces in robot-assisted surgery, see the surveys by Staub et al. [282] and Simorov et al. [283].

There are four different modes of endoscope positioning in the knowledge-based system: static, manual control, hands-on and autonom-

---

[8]See the remarks on the topic of "natural" human perception and machine sensing in 1.2.

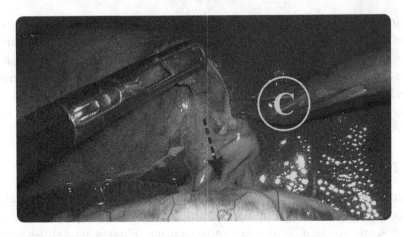

Figure 6.14: Illustration of two different manual repositionings of the endoscope intended by the surgeon. The circle indicates the intention to center the endoscopic view on the right instrument tip. The arrow denotes change of the perspective based on an anatomical landmark. Because instrument tips are known to the system, a symbolic interface is well suited to convey the surgeon's intention to the system. The anatomical landmark does not carry a distinct name and thus a subsymbolic interface is better suited.

ous. These can be selected either by voice control or through a web-based interface that can be used from a tablet, a smartphone or other touchscreen device. For manual control, a voice command interface, a foot pedal or a touch-based interface are implemented (cf. Fig.3.9).

6.3 Optional Action Components

The final part of the intraoperative system are optional action components. These are added on top of the autonomous endoscope guidance behavior to provide complementary features. Two specific action components are summarized in this section.

6.3.1 Extended Field of View through Live Stitching

One optional action component is extension of the field of view made possible by a slow continuous motion of the endoscope. Building on previous research on real-time[9] stitching or mosaicking [284][285] for endoscopic videos, I developed a solution that utilizes the knowledge that the endoscope is positioned by a robot [286]. The general idea of making use of the position information given by the endoscope robot has already been described by Vogt et al. [287]. However, the original approach was too slow for processing 30 images per second.

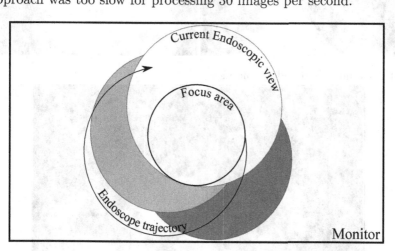

Figure 6.15: Visual radar metaphor to distinguish current from past information that comprises the extended field of view.

The field of view provided by endoscopes is often quite narrow, this can easily lead to a loss of anatomical orientation because of the missing visual context. To compensate, the endoscope is frequently repositioned to regain orientation, which leads to many unnecessary camera motions. Instead I propose a real-time stitching pipeline that continuously extends the field of view by continuous motion of the endoscope with GPU-based image postprocessing that shows a

---

[9]Here, as before in rendering, real-time simply means fast enough to process the sensor stream and is not related to real-time systems.

steady image to the surgeon. The unmodified live endoscope view is
embedded in a larger visual context, which is slowly updated.

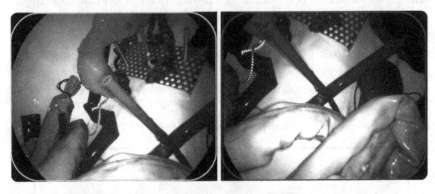

(a) Two individual endoscopic views.

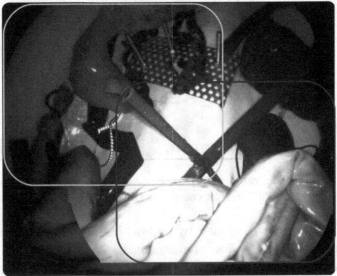

(b) Images combined into an extended field of view.

Figure 6.16: Results of the optional action component that extends the
field of view by live image stitching.

A radar display was used as visual metaphor to clearly show the respective age of each area in the resulting composite image (Fig. 6.15). The whole composite image is desaturated, blurred and faded out with each new camera image. This is done in order to avoid a situation where the surgeon erroneously perceives parts of the visual context as live image. In Fig. 6.16a two different individual endoscopic views into a box trainer are shown. Although there are significant landmarks in the scene, it is not directly obvious how the left and right image are spatially related. In contrast the extended view (Fig. 6.16b) does not only show the live image (to the lower right), but also further visual context for better orientation. .

6.3.2 Optimization of Redundant Degree of Freedom

The KUKA LWR IV has seven degrees of freedom and is thus kinematically redundant (cf. 4.2.4). By default, the unified Cartesian (cf. Fig. 4.7) and trocar (Fig. 6.10) interfaces do not expose this detail. In this case the position of the redundant DoF, or nullspace, is either fixed or positioning with all seven DoFs is used with an optimality criterion based on the inverse kinematics[10]. However, optional orthogonal interfaces are implemented in the platform that allow access to features not present in the unified ones. For the LWR this interface allows to move the robot's "elbow" on a circle independently of the flange position. As illustrated in Fig. 6.17, different places at the OR table are blocked depending on the setting for the redundant DoF. This can be deployed to make room for the surgical instruments in different phases of the intervention and to allow better access to the patient by OR staff – without disturbing endoscope positioning.

Adjustment of the redundant DoF can either be achieved by manual control or through utilization of other subsystems in the modular platform (cf. chapter 4). For manual control either voice commands or the web-based interface, e.g. on a tablet computer, can be used. Furthermore, due to the torque sensors integrated in each joint of the

---

[10]The analytical kinematics and nullspace optimization have been developed by Mirko Kunze.

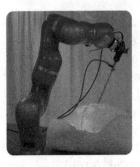 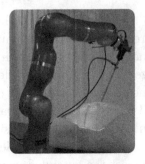 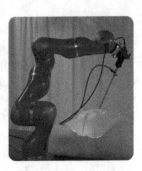

Figure 6.17: Optimization of a redundant degree of freedom during endoscope guidance for the LWR.

LWR, the elbow can also be used by direct interaction, i.e. pushing against the elbow, which only changes the elbow position without influence on the endoscope position. Automatic optimization utilizes the ceiling mounted RGB-D cameras to move the elbow as far away from all humans in the OR scene as possible. In automatic mode the nullspace is optimized using gradient descent on a weighted cost function in order to avoid joint limits and singularities and to maximize the distance to the closest object that is captured by cameras.

7 Evaluation Studies

All parts of the knowledge-based endoscope guidance system have been described in the previous chapters: System architecture, modular platform, tracking of surgical instruments, learning of endoscope guidance know-how and intraoperative robot-based action. In this chapter the evaluation results of the system in a phantom study of laparoscopic rectal resection with total mesorectal resection (TME) are provided. Starting from n=20 human assisted interventions, overall n=16 robot-assisted interventions were undertaken by one surgeon. Two robots with very different structure, the ViKY (2.1.9) and the LWR (4.2.4), have been used to position the endoscope. Learned know-how, in form of the camera quality classifiers (CQC), was acquired from both the human assistant and assistance of another robot. Average intervention duration for robot-assisted trials with the final CQC model was on the same level as with human assistance. The percentage of endoscopic views assessed with "good" in the robot-assisted interventions was found to be higher than with human assistance. Further objective measures are reported, such as length of instrument and endoscope trajectories.

One particular problem for evaluation of the knowledge-based camera guidance system has been hinted at in section 5.3.5. The intraoperative performance of the robot cannot be measured independently of expert judgement. Running the camera quality classifier on recorded interventions and comparing the classification of positions with the annotation is a valuable tool for investigation. Yet, the evaluation aims to assess the intraoperative quality of endoscopic views over time. This point can be made quite clear with an example: If the camera guidance is programmed to simply positioning the endoscope in the exact same position at the exact same times as recorded in the interventions, offline evaluation would consider the performance to be perfect. However, the intraoperative performance would be very poor. Therefore, evaluation of autonomous camera guidance is an interdisciplinary effort between surgeon and roboticist.

7.1 Metrics for Objective Assessment of Surgical Tasks

Apart from total intervention time T and assessment of relative camera quality Q, further measures known from literature can be applied. Satava et al. [288] provides an overview of objective metrics in 2003, these include

- Path length: $P = \sum_{0 < t \leq T} \sqrt{\|p_{t+1} - p_t\|}$ with $p \in \mathcal{P}$ being the positions of the instruments over time (usually recorded with a fixed $h = \Delta t = t_{i+1} - t_i$).

- Economy of movement (EOM): P/T

- Absence of motion (indecision): $I = \sum_t s(p_t)$
  $$\text{with } s(p_t) = \begin{cases} h & \|p_{t+1} - p_t\| < \tau \\ 0 & \text{otherwise} \end{cases}$$
  with τ being a velocity threshold close to zero.

- Purposefulness of motion

- Force measurements

- Counting of errors in different categories

From the paper by Oropesa et al. [289] published in 2011 two further criteria are

- Motion smoothness: $J = \sqrt{\frac{1}{2} \sum_t \|j\|^2}$ with jerk $j = \frac{\Delta_h^3 [p]}{h^3}$ (change of acceleration)

- Volume: $V = (\max_p \mathcal{P}) - (\min_p \mathcal{P})$

More information on objective skill assessment can be found in the review by Reiley et al. [290] from 2011. A collection of further criteria directly computable from a recorded trajectory is described by Weede et al. [291] in 2014.

Some of the above mentioned criteria will be used to compare the interventions with camera assistance by human or robot. However, while all of these criteria have been used (in combination) to distinguish novices from experts[1], not all criteria have a monotonic relationship between their numerical value and a notion of better. Intervention time T, path length P of instruments/endoscope and camera quality Q have a clear relationship between their numerical value and "better" and have thus been used in the following.

7.2 Experimental Setup

This section briefly provides same background on the experimental setup for the phantom study.

7.2.1 OpenHELP

The Open-Source Heidelberg Laparoscopic Phantom (OpenHELP) [292] is a medical phantom with realistic anatomy (Fig. 7.1) The torso is made out of plastic and different silicones are used for the organs to improve their haptic realism. All parts are based on a male CT scan.

Depending on the requirements of the scenario either a rigid abdominal wall can be used or a flexible one that allows to create a pneumoperitoneum. In the phantom study described here, the rigid abdominal wall[2] was chosen for ease of use. Furthermore, the phantom was extended for the specific intervention type by Mietkowski [293].

---

[1]See the discussion about construct validity in section 4.3.2.
[2]The rigid abdominal wall can be seen in Fig. 2.16a on p. 45.

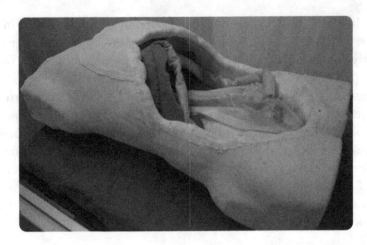

Figure 7.1: The Open-Source Heidelberg Laparoscopic Phantom (Open-HELP). For each intervention the phantom is equipped with a fresh set of connective tissue made out of latex and cords as vessels.

7.2.2 Laparoscopic Rectal Resection with Total Mesorectal Resection

A phantom model of laparoscopic rectal resection with total mesorectal resection was developed for the OpenHELP [294]. It consists of five phases (Fig. 7.2) with a total of 15 surgical steps. This intervention was chosen because it covers three quadrants in the abdomen and includes a variety of tasks and surgical instruments. Furthermore, camera guidance in the lesser pelvis is challenging due to the deep endoscope insertion and tight space.

Each intervention takes on the order of 25 minutes. Afterwards the cut latex cloths (connective tissue) and cords (vessels) have to be replaced (Fig. 7.3), which takes about 15 minutes.

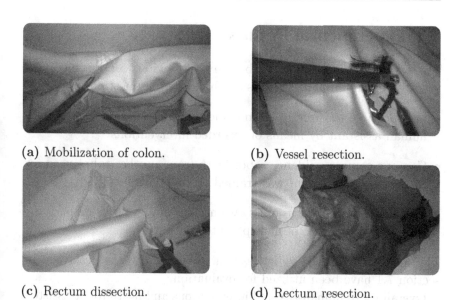

(a) Mobilization of colon.

(b) Vessel resection.

(c) Rectum dissection.

(d) Rectum resection.

Figure 7.2: Four major phases of the phantom intervention model. The first phase is diagnostic laparoscopy.

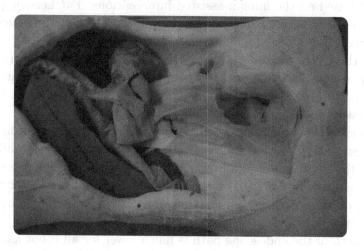

Figure 7.3: View into the OpenHELP after laparoscopic rectal resection with total mesorectal resection.

7.3 Experimental Results

The experimental setup described in the previous section has been used to get preliminary answers on the following questions:

• Is it possible to directly learn camera guidance know-how from a human assistant by means of recorded interventions?

• Can one camera guidance robot learn from another robot used for camera assistance that was trained on different data?

• Can the system learn from its own actions and improve its performance over the course of multiple interventions?

The metrics for objective assessment of surgical tasks described in section 7.1 have been utilized for evaluation.

Overall n=20 human-assisted interventions and n=16 robot-assisted ones have been performed. In Fig. 7.4 the structure of the experiments is shown. Five interventions each were performed on the ViKY and the LWR based on the human-assisted interventions. Furthermore, five interventions with the LWR were performed, which were trained on the five ViKY-assisted interventions. Finally, one trial was performed with the LWR trained on its ten previous interventions. An early report on the phantom series has been jointly published by the surgeon that performed the experiments and myself [295]. The preliminary analysis is shown on the following pages.

As can be seen in Fig. 7.5 there was a learning curve during the conventionally assisted interventions. Intervention times stabilized after the sixth trial. While the total duration was higher for the robot-assisted trials based on the human-assisted datasets, later trials based on the robot-assisted training datasets were superior to human assistance (Fig. 7.6).

Length of the endoscope path is much lower for all robot-assisted experiment groups (Fig. 7.8). However, the path length of the surgical instruments is higher for robotic endoscope guidance (Fig. 7.7). While the difference is large in early trials, for the later trials the

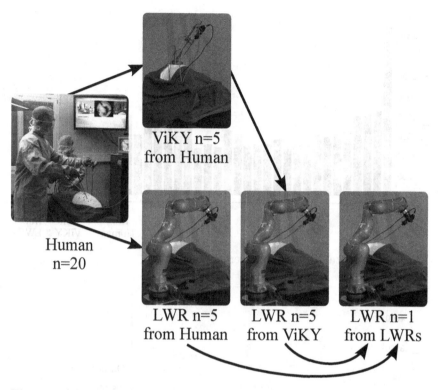

Figure 7.4: Phantom evaluation series. Human-to-Robot: Based on
n=20 human-assisted interventions, n=5 interventions were
assisted by the ViKY and n=5 by the LWR. Robot-to-Robot:
Afterwards, n=5 further LWR-assisted interventions were
performed only using the recorded ViKY trials as training
data. Finally, n=1 intervention was performed with the
LWR trained on its previous trials.

distances are nearly on the same level as for human assistance. A
plausible explanation is that the surgeon tried to correct poor views
in autonomous mode by servoing the robot to a better position. This
will be further investigated in later evaluations.

In Fig. 7.9 the ratio of different control modes is shown. During
the first ten robot-assisted trials, whose camera quality classifier was

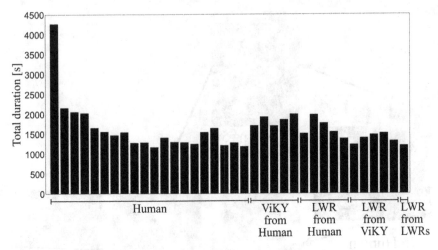

Figure 7.5: Total duration of interventions.

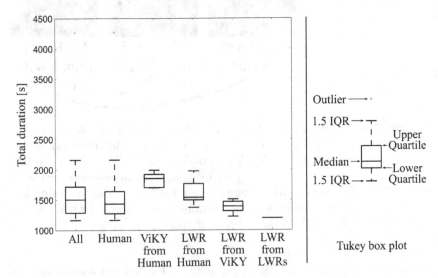

Figure 7.6: Tukey box plots for the total duration grouped by assistance and training data.

trained from the human-assisted recordings, a significant amount of manual robot control (24.7%) was necessary. In contrast, in the later

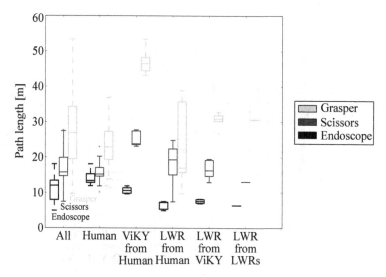

Figure 7.7: Grouped path length for grasper, scissors and endoscope.

six trials, only 6.3% were required. The same effect can be seen with respect to the camera quality. This difference is largely attributed to the improved recording system for the robot-assisted interventions, which recorded at a higher rate and with less instrument tracking occlusions.

The ratio of camera quality is the most direct criteria for the endoscope positioning performance. The "good" endoscopic views occur more often in all robot-assisted interventions compared to human assistance. Yet, only in case of the later six trials three conditions hold together: the average "good" ratio is higher, the variance between interventions is smaller and the "poor" positions occur far less.

Overall, for the six trials with the better training data, average intervention duration was 1290 seconds compared to 1626 seconds for human assistance. Furthermore, the endoscopic view was annotated as "good" to 52.8% for the robot-assisted interventions compared to only 27.8% with the human camera assistant. The autonomous mode was active 86.5% of the time. In conclusion, the knowledge-

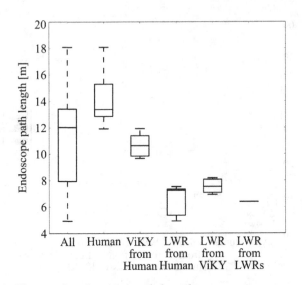

Figure 7.8: Grouped endoscope path length.

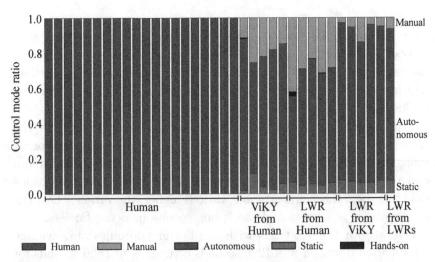

Figure 7.9: Ratio of endoscope control modes during the experiments.

based camera guidance system was found to be superior to the human camera assistant in the phantom study.

8 Conclusion

8.1 Discussion

The knowledge-based approach to autonomous endoscope positioning showed good performance in a complex phantom study. As shown in the previous chapter, in this study of overall n=36 interventions of about 25 minutes each, the system described in this thesis was actually superior to human camera assistance. Intervention duration was lower and the endoscopic view was considered good more often. Furthermore, the surgeon's load only increased slightly as the system was positioning the endoscope fully autonomous over 85% of the time. However, it must be cautioned that at this point in time no solid predictions can be made how well these positive results will carry over into clinical use. A study of cholecystectomy on pigs has been started, which is the next step after the presented phantom study towards clinical trials. Furthermore, a detailed journal article is in progress that will assess the presented system with an emphasis on the surgical point of view.

The modular platform (chapter 4) enabled evaluation of the system on two different robots that significantly differ in their kinematics. Thus, it was possible not only to evaluate whether the system can learn the endoscope guidance know-how from a human assistant, but also whether learning from another assisting robot is possible. Furthermore, several features of the platform facilitated research. First of all, the ability to add custom live visualizations and to introspect the overall system state proofed to be invaluable. Having a comprehensive simulation environment that allows to (automatically) test changes without requiring access to the real lab setup resulted in much quicker development iterations. The ability for loosely coupled development of subsystems provided the opportunity for synergies across research projects.

Relying on a knowledge-based architecture (chapter 3) results in a system that can be adapted for different types of surgical interventions, or preferences of the surgeon, without modifying its program code. The generic intraoperative action (chapter 6) component loads the learned camera guidance know-how (chapter 5) in form of phase-specific camera quality classifier (CQC). All specific robot motions, i.e. positioning of the endoscope relative to the instruments, solely originates from the learned model. No manual tweaks are required for different surgical tasks. Instead their characteristics are directly captured by the CQC.

Compared to the state of the art in endoscope holders and auto-mated camera positioning (chapter 2) two properties of the novel approach presented in this work stand out:

- No simple, constant and task-independent spatial relation between endoscope and instruments is assumed to be optimal. Instead the (minute) varieties present in the action of a good human camera assistant are captured in a dynamic model.

- Using the proposed classification for camera automation, even the approaches in the most advanced category, model-based planned and context-aware (class 8 in Fig. 2.39), make problematic assumptions. They either assume positioning know-how is available as factual knowledge and can be manually modeled or they require the surgeon to strictly follow a minutely detailed workflow. Instead the presented system only presupposes that the surgeon can judge whether an endoscopic view is suitable or not and that the intervention can by coarsely partitioned in surgical steps.

In the extensive survey on motorized endoscope holders, more than 25 custom-built kinematics, developed for endoscope guidance, have been identified in the literature. However, the question remains open, which is the best suited one with respect to its endoscope positioning performance in the OR. By adding a simple external interface to any of these endoscope positioning robots, all of them could be evaluated with the unmodified knowledge-based system.

To go beyond the current practical impact of over 20 years research into endoscope positioning, including several commercially available systems, a more extensive comparative evaluation is necessary. The systems of different groups should be compared to each other in a standard (animal) intervention model. Evaluation should be ideally performed by experts not involved into the development of the system. Different control modes, if available, should be compared, too. Objective metrics (cf. 7.1) should be agreed upon and utilized as benchmark. Otherwise, the current state of affairs, visible in chapter 2, will remain as it is today, many systems are developed and published, but no clear direction of progress becomes visible.

8.2 Future Work

There are three directions for future work on the autonomous endoscope guidance system.

First, evaluation of the system as in the phantom model (chapter 7), but with multiple surgeons and in an animal study of cholecystectomy on pigs. The only change to the system will occur in the knowledge base by replacing the CQC models with ones trained for cholecystectomy. At the time of writing, seven pig cholecystectomies with a human camera assistant have been recorded and are currently annotated with endoscopic view quality for training.

Second, the presented system directly derives its endoscope positioning behavior from observations of a human camera assistant. Yet, the factual (textbook) knowledge on endoscope guidance, e.g. keeping the horizon stable and complying to the trocar constraint, were manually determined by a procedural program. Developing further what has been said about knowledge-based systems (cf. 1.3), the next step is to automatically derive these contextual conditions for the assistance function from the knowledge base. For example, an ontology combined with a reasoner could be deployed to achieve this objective. Thereby, a possible progression from manually controlled endoscope positioning systems to learned autonomous ones – as presented here ($\star$) – could be continued to reasoning-based autonomy that uses learned models for subtasks:

Manual control $\Rightarrow$ Programmed Automatons

$\Rightarrow$ Programmed Autonomous Robots

$\Rightarrow$ Learned Task-specific Autonomy ($\star$)

$\Rightarrow$ Reasoning-based Autonomy (with learned subtaks)

Third, apply the method of adaptive sampling of forward classifiers (cf. 5.3 & 6.2) to other tasks in (surgical) robotics. A relatively straight forward transfer of the adaptive-sampling-of-classifier approach are further handling tasks in (minimally-invasive) surgery that are quasi-static in their physical dynamics. For these applicability is largely a question of whether the classifier model can be trained well. Deriving action from these models can be very similar to the one presented here. Finally, given the high number of samples that can be evaluated on modern computer hardware, the most interesting application would be to robotic tasks with significant dynamics.

Bibliography

[1] E. Mühe. Die erste cholecystektomie durch das laparoskop. *Langenbecks Archiv Für Chirurgie*, 369(1):804, 1986. Cited on page(s): 2

[2] Alfred Cuschieri, Francois Dubois, Jean Mouiel, Phillipe Mouret, Hans Becker, Gerhardt Buess, Michael Trede, and Hans Troidl. The european experience with laparoscopic cholecystectomy. *The American Journal of Surgery*, 161(3):385 – 387, 1991. Cited on page(s): 3

[3] Judy A Shea, Michael J Healey, Jesse A Berlin, John R Clarke, Peter F Malet, Rudolf N Staroscik, J Sanford Schwartz, and Sankey V Williams. Mortality and complications associated with laparoscopic cholecystectomy. a meta-analysis. *Annals of Surgery*, 224(5):609–620, 1996. Cited on page(s): 3

[4] W. Y. Lau, C. K. Leow, and A. K. C. Li. History of endoscopic and laparoscopic surgery. *World Journal of Surgery*, 21(4):444–453, 1997. Cited on page(s): 3

[5] P Breedveld, HG Stassen, DW Meijer, and LPS Stassen. Theoretical background and conceptual solution for depth perception and eye-hand coordination problems in laparoscopic surgery. *Minimally Invasive Therapy & Allied Technologies*, 8(4):227–234, 1999. Cited on page(s): 4

[6] P. Breedveld and M. Wentink. Eye-hand coordination in laparoscopy - an overview of experiments and supporting aids. *Minimally Invasive Therapy and Allied Technologies*, 10(3):155–162, 2001. Cited on page(s): 4

[7] J. Dankelman, M. K. Chmarra, E. G. G. Verdaasdonk, L. P. S. Stassen, and C. A. Grimbergen. Fundamental aspects of learning minimally invasive surgical skills. *Minimally Invasive Therapy & Allied Technologies*, 14:247–256, 2005. Cited on page(s): 4

[8] H. G. Stassen, J. Dankelman, and C. A. Grimbergen. Open versus minimally invasive surgery: a man-machine system approach. *Transactions of the Institute of Measurement and Control*, 21:151–162, 1999. Cited on page(s): 4, 7

[9] AG Gallagher, N McClure, J McGuigan, K Ritchie, and NP Sheehy. An ergonomic analysis of the fulcrum effect in the acquisition of endoscopic skills. *Endoscopy*, 30(7):617–620, 1998. Cited on page(s): 4

[10] Bin Zheng, MariaA. Cassera, DannyV. Martinec, GeorgO. Spaun, and LeeL. Swanström. Measuring mental workload during the performance of advanced laparoscopic tasks. *Surgical Endoscopy*, 24(1):45–50, 2010. Cited on page(s): 4

[11] E. Matt Ritter and Daniel J. Scott. Design of a proficiency-based skills training curriculum for the fundamentals of laparoscopic surgery. *Surgical Innovation*, 14(2):107–112, 2007. Cited on page(s): 4, 98

[12] MJ Van Det, WJHJ Meijerink, C Hoff, ER Totte, and JPEN Pierie. Optimal ergonomics for laparoscopic surgery in minimally invasive surgery suites: a review and guidelines. *Surgical endoscopy*, 23(6):1279–1285, 2009. Cited on page(s): 6

[13] LSGL Wauben, MA Van Veelen, D Gossot, and RHM Goossens. Application of ergonomic guidelines during minimally invasive surgery: a questionnaire survey of 284 surgeons. *Surgical Endoscopy And Other Interventional Techniques*, 20(8):1268–1274, 2006. Cited on page(s): 6

[14] E. C. Lee, A. Rafiq, R. Merrell, R. Ackerman, and J. T. Dennerlein. Ergonomics and human factors in endoscopic surgery: a

comparison of manual vs telerobotic simulation systems. *Surgical Endoscopy And Other Interventional Techniques*, 19(8):1064–1070, 2005. Cited on page(s): 6

[15] Ulrich Matern and Sonja Koneczny. Safety, hazards and ergonomics in the operating room. *Surgical Endoscopy*, 21(11):1965–1969, 2007. Cited on page(s): 6

[16] Gyusung Lee, Tommy Lee, David Dexter, Carlos Godinez, Nora Meenaghan, Robert Catania, and Adrian Park. Ergonomic risk associated with assisting in minimally invasive surgery. *Surgical endoscopy*, 23(1):182–188, 2009. Cited on page(s): 6

[17] MICHAEL E MORAN. Stationary and automated laparoscopically assisted technologies. *Journal of Laparoendoscopic Surgery*, 3(3):221–227, 1993. Cited on page(s): 6, 24

[18] GB Hanna, S Shimi, and A Cuschieri. Influence of direction of view, target-to-endoscope distance and manipulation angle on endoscopic knot tying. *British journal of surgery*, 84(10):1460–1464, 1997. Cited on page(s): 7, 8

[19] George B Hanna, Sami M Shimi, and Alfred Cuschieri. Task performance in endoscopic surgery is influenced by location of the image display. *Annals of Surgery*, 227(4):481–484, 1998. Cited on page(s): 7, 8

[20] G. B. Hanna and A. Cuschieri. Influence of the optical axis-to-target view angle on endoscopic task performance. *Surgical Endoscopy*, 13(4):371–375, 1999. Cited on page(s): 8

[21] P. V. Patil, G. B. Hanna, and A. Cuschieri. Effect of the angle between the optical axis of the endoscope and the instruments' plane on monitor image and surgical performance. *Surgical Endoscopy And Other Interventional Techniques*, 18(1):111–114, 2004. Cited on page(s): 8

[22] T. A. Emam, G. Hanna, and A. Cuschieri. Ergonomic principles of task alignment, visual display, and direction of execution of laparoscopic bowel suturing. *Surgical Endoscopy And Other Interventional Techniques*, 16(2):267–271, 2002. Cited on page(s): 9

[23] F. Voorhorst, D. Meijer, C. Overbeeke, and G. Smets. Depth perception in laparoscopy through perception-action coupling. *Minimally Invasive Therapy & Allied Technologies*, 7(4):325–334, 1998. Cited on page(s): 9

[24] LK Jacobs, V Shayani, and JM Sackier. Determination of the learning curve of the aesop robot. *Surgical endoscopy*, 11(1):54–55, 1997. Cited on page(s): 9, 27, 73

[25] Stephen B Shew, Daniel J Ostlie, and George W Holcomb III. Robotic telescopic assistance in pediatric laparoscopic surgery. *Pediatric Endosurgery and Innovative Techniques*, 7(4):371–376, 2003. Cited on page(s): 9, 24, 28, 73

[26] Yohannes Kassahun, Bingbin Yu, AbrahamTemesgen Tibebu, Danail Stoyanov, Stamatia Giannarou, JanHendrik Metzen, and Emmanuel Vander Poorten. Surgical robotics beyond enhanced dexterity instrumentation: a survey of machine learning techniques and their role in intelligent and autonomous surgical actions. *International Journal of Computer Assisted Radiology and Surgery*, pages 1–16, 2015. Cited on page(s): 10, 158

[27] Martin Hägele, Klas Nilsson, and J Norberto Pires. Industrial robotics. In *Springer handbook of robotics*, pages 963–986. Springer, 2008. Cited on page(s): 10

[28] Heidi Ryan and Shawn Tsuda. History of and current systems in robotic surgery. In Matthew Kroh and Sricharan Chalikonda, editors, *Essentials of Robotic Surgery*, pages 1–12. Springer International Publishing, 2015. Cited on page(s): 10

[29] F. Pugin, P. Bucher, and P. Morel. History of robotic surgery: From aesop and zeus to da vinci. *Journal of Visceral Surgery*, 1485:e3 – e8, 2011. Cited on page(s): 10

[30] Satyam Kalan, Sanket Chauhan, RafaelF. Coelho, MarceloA. Orvieto, IgnacioR. Camacho, KennethJ. Palmer, and VipulR. Patel. History of robotic surgery. *Journal of Robotic Surgery*, 4(3):141–147, 2010. Cited on page(s): 10

[31] Douglas R. Ewing, Alessio Pigazzi, Yulun Wang, and Garth H. Ballantyne. Robots in the operating room - the history. *Surgical Innovation*, 11(2):63–71, 2004. Cited on page(s): 10

[32] N. G. Hockstein, C. G. Gourin, R. A. Faust, and D. J. Terris. A history of robots: from science fiction to surgical robotics. *Journal of Robotic Surgery*, 1(2):113–118, 2007. Cited on page(s): 12

[33] Simon DiMaio, Mike Hanuschik, and Usha Kreaden. The da vinci surgical system. In Jacob Rosen, Blake Hannaford, and Richard M. Satava, editors, *Surgical Robotics*, pages 199–217. Springer US, 2011. Cited on page(s): 12, 69

[34] H. G. Kenngott, L. Fischer, F. Nickel, J. Rom, J. Rassweiler, and B. P. Müller-Stich. Status of robotic assistance - a less traumatic and more accurate minimally invasive surgery? *Langenbeck's Archives of Surgery*, 397(3):333–341, 2012. Cited on page(s): 12

[35] Ulrich Hagn, R. Konietschke, A. Tobergte, M. Nickl, S. Jörg, B. Kübler, G. Passig, M. Gröger, F. Fröhlich, U. Seibold, L. Le-Tien, A. Albu-Schäffer, A. Nothhelfer, F. Hacker, M. Grebenstein, and G. Hirzinger. Dlr mirosurge: a versatile system for research in endoscopic telesurgery. *International Journal of Computer Assisted Radiology and Surgery*, 5(2):183–193, 2010. Cited on page(s): 12, 69

[36] G. P. Moustris, S. C. Hiridis, K. M. Deliparaschos, and K. M. Konstantinidis. Evolution of autonomous and semi-autonomous

robotic surgical systems: a review of the literature. *The International Journal of Medical Robotics and Computer Assisted Surgery*, 7(4), 2011. Cited on page(s): 12, 14

[37] William L Bargar, André Bauer, and Martin Börner. Primary and revision total hip replacement using the robodoc (r) system. *Clinical Orthopaedics and Related Research*, 354:82–91, 1998. Cited on page(s): 13

[38] Benny Hagag, Rony Abovitz, Hyosig Kang, Brian Schmitz, and Michael Conditt. Rio: Robotic-arm interactive orthopedic system makoplasty: User interactive haptic orthopedic robotics. In Jacob Rosen, Blake Hannaford, and Richard M. Satava, editors, *Surgical Robotics*, pages 219–246. Springer US, 2011. Cited on page(s): 13

[39] John R Adler Jr, SD Chang, MJ Murphy, J Doty, P Geis, and SL Hancock. The cyberknife: a frameless robotic system for radiosurgery. *Stereotactic and Functional Neurosurgery*, 69:124–128, 1997. Cited on page(s): 14

[40] Mathias Hoeckelmann, Imre J Rudas, Paolo Fiorini, Frank Kirchner, and Tamas Haidegger. Current capabilities and development potential in surgical robotics. *Int J Adv Robot Syst*, 12:1–39, 2015. Cited on page(s): 17

[41] Ryu Nakadate, Jumpei Arata, and Makoto Hashizume. Next-generation robotic surgery - from the aspect of surgical robots developed by industry. *Minimally Invasive Therapy & Allied Technologies*, 24(1):2–7, 2015. Cited on page(s): 17

[42] St. Erbse, K. Radermacher, M. Anton, G. Rau, W. Boeckmann, G. Jakse, and H. W. Staudte. Development of an automatic surgical holding system based on ergonomic analysis. In Jocelyne Troccaz, Eric Grimson, and Ralph Mösges, editors, *CVRMed-MRCAS'97*, volume 1205 of *Lecture Notes in Computer Science*,

pages 737–746. Springer Berlin Heidelberg, 1997. Cited on page(s): 23

[43] Matthias Winkler, Stephan Erbse, Klaus Radermacher, Günter Rau, and Werner Rath. An automatic camera-holding system for gynecologic laparoscopy. *The Journal of the American Association of Gynecologic Laparoscopists*, 8(2):303 – 306, 2001. Cited on page(s): 23

[44] M. O. Schurr, A. Arezzo, B. Neisius, H. Rininsland, H. U. Hilzinger, J. Dorn, K. Roth, and G. F. Buess. Trocar and instrument positioning system tiska. *Surgical Endoscopy*, 13(5):528–531, 1999. Cited on page(s): 24

[45] A. Grimbergen, J. E. N Jaspers, J. L Herder, and H. G Stassen. Development of laparoscopic instruments. *Minimally Invasive Therapy & Allied Technologies*, 10(3):145–154, 2001. Cited on page(s): 24

[46] T. Kimura, Y. Umehara, and S. Matsumoto. Laparoscopic cholecystectomy performed by a single surgeon using a visual field tracking camera. *Surgical Endoscopy*, 14(9):825–829, 2000. Cited on page(s): 24

[47] H. Niebuhr and O. Born. Image tracking system eine neue technik für die sichere und kostensparende laparoskopische operation. *Der Chirurg*, 71(5):580–584, 2000. Cited on page(s): 24

[48] Jonathan Kim, Yun-Ju Lee, Seong-Young Ko, Dong-Soo Kwon, and Woo-Jung Lee. Compact camera assistant robot for minimally invasive surgery: Kalar. In *Intelligent Robots and Systems, 2004.(IROS 2004). Proceedings. 2004 IEEE/RSJ International Conference on*, volume 3, pages 2587–2592. IEEE, 2004. Cited on page(s): 24

[49] Seong-Young Ko, Jonathan Kim, Woo-Jung Lee, and Dong-Soo Kwon. Compact laparoscopic assistant robot using a bending

mechanism. *Advanced Robotics*, 21:689–709, 2007. Cited on page(s): 24

[50] Ren C. Luo, Jui Wang, Chih Kang Chang, and Yi Wen Perng. Surgeon's third hand: An assistive robot endoscopic system with intuitive maneuverability for laparoscopic surgery. In *Biomedical Robotics and Biomechatronics (2014 5th IEEE RAS EMBS International Conference on*, pages 138–143, Aug 2014. Cited on page(s): 24

[51] Brahim Tamadazte, Anthony Agustinos, Philippe Cinquin, Gaelle Fiard, and Sandrine Voros. Multi-view vision system for laparoscopy surgery. *International Journal of Computer Assisted Radiology and Surgery*, 10(2):195–203, 2015. Cited on page(s): 24

[52] A. Arezzo, F. Ulmer, O. Weiss, M. O. Schurr, M. Hamad, and G. F. Buess. Experimental trial on solo surgery for minimally invasive therapy. *Surgical Endoscopy*, 14(10):955–959, 2000. Cited on page(s): 24, 27, 73

[53] Malcolm G. Munro. Automated laparoscope positioner: Preliminary experience. *The Journal of the American Association of Gynecologic Laparoscopists*, 1(1):67 – 70, 1993. Cited on page(s): 25, 73

[54] J. M. Sackier and Y. Wang. Robotically assisted laparoscopic surgery. *Surgical Endoscopy*, 8(1):63–66, 1994. Cited on page(s): 26, 73

[55] G.H. Ballantyne. Robotic surgery, telerobotic surgery, telepresence, and telementoring. *Surgical Endoscopy And Other Interventional Techniques*, 16(10):1389–1402, 2002. Cited on page(s): 26, 28, 29, 73

[56] Yulun Wang and Keith Phillip Laby. Automated endoscope system for optimal positioning, May 25 1999. US Patent 5,907,664. Cited on page(s): 27, 73

[57] M. E. Allaf, S. V. Jackman, P. G. Schulam, J. A. Cadeddu, B. R. Lee, R. G. Moore, and L. R. Kavoussi. Laparoscopic visual field. *Surgical Endoscopy*, 12(12):1415–1418, 1998. Cited on page(s): 27, 73

[58] AW Partin, JB Adams, RG Moore, and LR Kavoussi. Complete robot-assisted laparoscopic urologic surgery: a preliminary report. *Journal of the American College of Surgeons*, 181(6):552–557, December 1995. Cited on page(s): 27, 73

[59] L Mettler, M Ibrahim, and W Jonat. One year of experience working with the aid of a robotic assistant (the voice-controlled optic holder aesop) in gynaecological endoscopic surgery. *Human Reproduction*, 13(10):2748–2750, 1998. Cited on page(s): 28, 73

[60] Louis R. Kavoussi, Robert G. Moore, John B. Adams, and Alan W. Partin. Comparison of robotic versus human laparoscopic camera control. *The Journal of Urology*, 154(6):2134 – 2136, 1995. Cited on page(s): 28, 73

[61] Pedro Ballester Nebot, Yatin Jain, Kevin Haylett, Robert Stone, and Rory McCloy. Comparison of task performance of the camera-holder robots endoassist and aesop. *Surgical Laparoscopy Endoscopy & Percutaneous Techniques*, 13(5):334–338, 2003. Cited on page(s): 28, 38, 73, 74

[62] Marius M. Punt, Coen N. Stefels, Cornelis A. Grimbergen, and Jenny Dankelman. Evaluation of voice control, touch panel control and assistant control during steering of an endoscope. *Minimally Invasive Therapy & Allied Technologies*, 14(3):181–187, 2005. Cited on page(s): 28

[63] K. Kipfmüller. The use of aesop 3000 in laparoscopic colon resection. *Minimally Invasive Therapy & Allied Technologies*, 9:327, 2000. Cited on page(s): 28

[64] Joaquim Fernando Martins Rua, Fabio Biscegli Jatene, José Ribas Milanez de Campos, Rosangela Monteiro, Miguel Lia

Tedde, Marcos Naoyuki Samano, Wanderley M. Bernardo, and João Carlos Das-Neves-Pereira. Robotic versus human camera holding in video-assisted thoracic sympathectomy: a single blind randomized trial of efficacy and safety. *Interactive CardioVascular and Thoracic Surgery*, 8(2):195–199, 2009. Cited on page(s): 28, 73

[65] Stephen Merola, Philip Weber, Annette Wasielewski, and Garth H Ballantyne. Comparison of laparoscopic colectomy with and without the aid of a robotic camera holder. *Surgical Laparoscopy Endoscopy & Percutaneous Techniques*, 12(1):46–51, 2002. Cited on page(s): 29, 73

[66] Jan Martin Proske, Ibrahim Dagher, and Dominique Franco. Comparative study of human and robotic camera control in laparoscopic biliary and colon surgery. *Journal of Laparoendoscopic & Advanced Surgical Techniques*, 14(6):345–348, 2004. Cited on page(s): 29

[67] B.M. Kraft, C. Jäger, K. Kraft, B.J. Leibl, and R. Bittner. The aesop robot system in laparoscopic surgery: Increased risk or advantage for surgeon and patient? *Surgical Endoscopy And Other Interventional Techniques*, 18(8):1216–1223, 2004. Cited on page(s): 29, 73

[68] R. Hurteau, S. DeSantis, E. Begin, and M. Gagner. Laparoscopic surgery assisted by a robotic cameraman: concept and experimental results. In *Robotics and Automation, 1994. Proceedings., 1994 IEEE International Conference on*, volume 3, pages 2286–2289, May 1994. Cited on page(s): 30, 73

[69] Eric Begin, Michel Gagner, Richard Hurteau, Sylvio de Santis, and Alfons Pomp. A robotic camera for laparoscopic surgery: conception and experimental results. *Surgical Laparoscopy Endoscopy & Percutaneous Techniques*, 5(1):6–11, 1995. Cited on page(s): 30, 73

[70] Michel Gagner, Eric Begin, Richard Hurteau, and Alfons Pomp. Robotic interactive laparoscopic cholecystectomy. *The Lancet*, 343(8897):596 – 597, 1994. Originally published as Volume 1, Issue 8897. Cited on page(s): 30

[71] Russell H Taylor, Janez Funda, Ben Eldridge, Steve Gomory, Kreg Gruben, David LaRose, Mark Talamini, Louis Kavoussi, and James Anderson. A telerobotic assistant for laparoscopic surgery. *Engineering in Medicine and Biology Magazine, IEEE*, 14(3):279–288, 1995. Cited on page(s): 31, 32, 73

[72] Janez Funda, B. N. Eldridge, Kreg Gruben, Steve Gomory, and Russell H. Taylor. Comparison of two manipulator designs for laparoscopic surgery. volume 2351, pages 172–183, 1995. Cited on page(s): 31, 34, 73

[73] J. Funda, R. H. Taylor, Benjamin Eldridge, S. Gomory, and K. G. Gruben. Constrained cartesian motion control for teleoperated surgical robots. *Robotics and Automation, IEEE Transactions on*, 12(3):453–465, Jun 1996. Cited on page(s): 32, 33, 73

[74] J. Funda, K. Gruben, B. Eldridge, S. Gomory, and R. Taylor. Control and evaluation of a 7-axis surgical robot for laparoscopy. In *Robotics and Automation, 1995. Proceedings., 1995 IEEE International Conference on*, volume 2, pages 1477–1484, May 1995. Cited on page(s): 33, 73

[75] N. J. Dowler and S. R. J. Holland. The evolutionary design of an endoscopic telemanipulator. *Robotics Automation Magazine, IEEE*, 3(4):38–45, Dec 1996. Cited on page(s): 35, 73

[76] Patrick A Finlay and Rory F McCloy. The endoassist endoscopic camera holder. *Primer of Robotic and Telerobotic Surgery*, pages 42–48, 2004. Cited on page(s): 35, 74

[77] SashiS. Kommu, Peter Rimington, Christopher Anderson, and Abhay Rané. Initial experience with the endoassist camera-holding robot in laparoscopic urological surgery. *Journal of*

Robotic Surgery, 1(2):133–137, 2007. Cited on page(s): 36, 37, 74

[78] Patrick A Finlay. A robotic camera holder for laparoscopy. In *Proceedings and Overviews of ICAR2001 Workshop*, volume 2, pages 129–132, 2001. Cited on page(s): 35, 37, 74

[79] FA Voorhorst, DW Meijer, and CJ Overbeeke. Head-controlled laparoscopy: Experiment, prototype, and preliminary results. *Journal of Laparoendoscopic & Advanced Surgical Techniques*, 9(5):379–388, 1999. Cited on page(s): 36

[80] He Su, Jianmin Li, Huaifeng Zhang, Jinhua Li, and Shuxin Wang. Using motion parallax for laparoscopic surgery. *The International Journal of Medical Robotics and Computer Assisted Surgery*, 2015. Cited on page(s): 36

[81] P. A. Finlay and M. H. Ornstein. Controlling the movement of a surgical laparoscope. *Engineering in Medicine and Biology Magazine, IEEE*, 14(3):289–291, May 1995. Cited on page(s): 37, 73

[82] PA Finlay. Clinical experience with a goniometric head-controlled laparoscope manipulator. In *Proc. IARP Workshop on Medical Robotics, Vienna*, 1996. Cited on page(s): 37, 73

[83] S Aiono, JM Gilbert, B Soin, PA Finlay, and A Gordan. Controlled trial of the introduction of a robotic camera assistant (endo assist) for laparoscopic cholecystectomy. *Surgical Endoscopy and Other Interventional Techniques*, 16(9):1267–1270, 2002. Cited on page(s): 37, 74

[84] Sashi S Kommu and Abhay Rané. Camera holding robotic devices in urology. In Vanja Bozovic, editor, *Medical Robotics*, chapter 25, pages 341–350. INTECH Open Access Publisher, Vienna, 1 edition, 2008. Cited on page(s): 37, 74

[85] Yunus Yavuz, Brynjulf Ystgaard, Eirik Skogvoll, and Ronald Mårvik. A comparative experimental study evaluating the performance of surgical robots aesop and endosista. *Surgical Laparoscopy Endoscopy & Percutaneous Techniques*, 10(3):163–167, 2000. Cited on page(s): 37, 73

[86] Andrew A. Wagner, Ioannis M. Varkarakis, Richard E. Link, Wendy Sullivan, and Li-Ming Su. Comparison of surgical performance during laparoscopic radical prostatectomy of two robotic camera holders, endoassist and aesop: A pilot study. *Urology*, 68(1):70 – 74, 2006. Cited on page(s): 38, 74

[87] K. T. Boer, M. Bruijn, J. E. Jaspers, L. P. S. Stassen, W. F. M. Erp, A. Jansen, P. M. N. Y. H. Go, J. Dankelman, and D. J. Gouma. Time-action analysis of instrument positioners in laparoscopic cholecystectomy. *Surgical Endoscopy And Other Interventional Techniques*, 16(1):142–147, 2002. Cited on page(s): 38, 73

[88] Marc O. Schurr, Alberto Arezzo, and Gerhard F. Buess. Robotics and systems technology for advanced endoscopic procedures: experiences in general surgery. *European Journal of Cardio-Thoracic Surgery*, 16:97–105, 1999. Cited on page(s): 38, 39, 74

[89] Hermann Rininsland. Artemis. a telemanipulator for cardiac surgery. *European Journal of Cardio-Thoracic Surgery*, 16:106–111, 1999. Cited on page(s): 39

[90] Hsiao-Wei Tang, H. Van Brussel, D. Reynaerts, J. Vander Sloten, and P. R. Koninckx. A laparoscopic robot with intuitive interface for gynecological laser laparoscopy. In *Robotics and Automation, 2003. Proceedings. ICRA '03. IEEE International Conference on*, volume 2, pages 2646–2650, Sept 2003. Cited on page(s): 39

[91] G. F. Buess, A. Arezzo, M. O. Schurr, F. Ulmer, H. Fisher, L. Gumb, T. Testa, and C. Nobman. A new remote-controlled

endoscope positioning system for endoscopic solo surgery. *Surgical Endoscopy*, 14(4):395–399, 2000. Cited on page(s): 39, 74

[92] Buess GF, Schurr MO, and Fischer SC. Robotics and allied technologies in endoscopic surgery. *Archives of Surgery*, 135(2):229–235, 2000. Cited on page(s): 40, 74

[93] A Arezzo, T Testa, F Ulmer, MO Schurr, M Degregori, and GF Buess. Positioning systems for endoscopic solo surgery. *Minerva Chirurgica*, 55(9):635–641, September 2000. Cited on page(s): 40, 74

[94] H. Fischer, M. Selig, J. Vagner, B. Vogel, E. Hempel, M. Kaiser, K. Brhel, A. Hinz, A. Felden, A. Schäf, L. Gumb, U. Ullrich, A. Grünhagen, U. Voges, H. Kühnapfel, H. Çakmak, H. Maass, H. Becker, H. Breitwieser, R. Mikut, R. Oberle, W. Eppler, P. Schlossmacher, W. Pfleging, W. A. Kaiser, S. Schüler, R. Cichon, M. Cornelius, U. Kappert, M. O. Schurr, G. Buess, and V. Falk. The medical engineering program of forschungszentrum karlsruhe. *Minimally Invasive Therapy & Allied Technologies*, 9:255–267, 2000. Cited on page(s): 40

[95] V. F. Munoz, C. Vara-Thorbeck, J. G. DeGabriel, J. F. Lozano, E. Sanchez-Badajoz, A. Garcia-Cerezo, R. Toscano, and A. Jimenez-Garrido. A medical robotic assistant for minimally invasive surgery. In *Robotics and Automation, 2000. Proceedings. ICRA '00. IEEE International Conference on*, volume 3, pages 2901–2906, 2000. Cited on page(s): 40, 74

[96] C. Vara-Thorbeck, V. F. Muñoz, R. Toscano, J. Gomez, J. Fernández, M. Felices, and A. Garcia-Cerezo. A new robotic endoscope manipulator. *Surgical Endoscopy*, 15(9):924–927, 2001. Cited on page(s): 41, 74

[97] Victor F. Muñoz, J. Fernández-Lozano, J. Gómez-de Gabriel, I. García-Morales, R. Molina Mesa, and C. Pérez-del Pulgar. On

laparoscopic robot design and validation. *Integrated Computer-Aided Engineering*, 10(3):211–229, 2003. Cited on page(s): 41, 74

[98] Victor F Munoz, J Gómez de Gabriel, J Fernández-Lozano, I Garcia-Morales, R Molina-Mesa, C Perez-del Pulgar, J Seron-Barba, and M Azouaghe. Design and control of a robotic assistant for laparoscopic surgery. In *International Symposium on Intelligent Robotic Systems*, pages 393–401, 2001. Cited on page(s): 41, 74

[99] J. Fernandez-Lozano, J. M. G. de Gabriel, V. F. Munoz, I. Garcia-Morales, D. Melgar, C. Vara, and A. Garcia-Cerezo. Human-machine interface evaluation in a computer assisted surgical system. In *Robotics and Automation, 2004. Proceedings. ICRA '04. 2004 IEEE International Conference on*, volume 1, pages 231–236, April 2004. Cited on page(s): 41, 74

[100] V. F. Muñoz, J. M. Gómez de Gabriel, I. García-Morales, J. Fernández-Lozano, and J. Morales. Pivoting motion control for a laparoscopic assistant robot and human clinical trials. *Advanced Robotics*, 19(6):694–712, 2005. Cited on page(s): 41, 74

[101] V. F. Muñoz, I. Garcia-Morales, C. Perez del Pulgar, J. M. Gomez-DeGabriel, J. Fernandez-Lozano, A. Garcia-Cerezo, C. Vara-Thorbeck, and R. Toscano. Control movement scheme based on manipulability concept for a surgical robotic assistant. In *Robotics and Automation, 2006. ICRA 2006. Proceedings 2006 IEEE International Conference on*, pages 245–250, May 2006. Cited on page(s): 42, 74

[102] P Berkelman, Philippe Cinquin, Jocelyne Troccaz, J Ayoubi, Christian Letoublon, and F Bouchard. A compact, compliant laparoscopic endoscope manipulator. In *Robotics and Automation, 2002. Proceedings. ICRA '02. IEEE International Conference on*,

238   *Bibliography*

volume 2, pages 1870–1875. IEEE, 2002. Cited on page(s): 42, 74

[103] PeterJ. Berkelman, Philippe Cinquin, Jocelyne Troccaz, Jean-Marc Ayoubi, and Christian Létoublon. Development of a compact cable-driven laparoscopic endoscope manipulator. In Takeyoshi Dohi and Ron Kikinis, editors, *Medical Image Computing and Computer-Assisted Intervention — MICCAI 2002*, volume 2488 of *Lecture Notes in Computer Science*, pages 17–24. Springer Berlin Heidelberg, 2002. Cited on page(s): 42, 74

[104] P. Berkelman, E. Boidard, P. Cinquin, and J. Troccaz. Ler: the light endoscope robot. In *Intelligent Robots and Systems, 2003. (IROS 2003). Proceedings. 2003 IEEE/RSJ International Conference on*, volume 3, pages 2835–2840, Oct 2003. Cited on page(s): 42, 74

[105] Jean-Alexandre Long, Philippe Cinquin, Jocelyne Troccaz, Jean-Jacques Rambeaud, Olivier Skowron, Peter Berkelman, Christian Letoublon, Pierre Cadi, Frédéric Bocqueraz, Sandrine Voros, and Jean-Luc Descotes. Preclinical development of the timc ler (light endoscope robot). *Progres En Urologie : Journal de L'Association Francaise D'urologie Et de La Societe Francaise D'urologie*, 16(1):45—51, February 2006. Cited on page(s): 43, 74

[106] Jean-Alexandre Long, Philippe Cinquin, Jocelyne Troccaz, Sandrine Voros, Peter Berkelman, Jean-Luc Descotes, Christian Letoublon, and Jean-Jacques Rambeaud. Development of miniaturized light endoscope-holder robot for laparoscopic surgery. *Journal of Endourology*, 21(8):911–914, 2007. Cited on page(s): 43, 74

[107] S. Voros, G. P. Haber, J. F. Menudet, J. A. Long, and P. Cinquin. Viky robotic scope holder: Initial clinical experience and preliminary results using instrument tracking. *Mechatronics*,

IEEE/ASME Transactions on, 15(6):879–886, Dec 2010. Cited on page(s): 43, 46, 74

[108] Andrew A Gumbs, Fernando Crovari, Clement Vidal, Patrick Henri, and Brice Gayet. Modified robotic lightweight endoscope (viky) validation in vivo in a porcine model. *Surgical Innovation*, 14(4):261–264, 2007. Cited on page(s): 43, 74

[109] Jean-Alexandre Long, Jacques Tostain, Cecilia Lanchon, Sandrine Voros, Maud Medici, Jean-Luc Descotes, Jocelyne Troccaz, Philippe Cinquin, Jean-Jacques Rambeaud, and Alexandre Moreau-Gaudry. First clinical experience in urologic surgery with a novel robotic lightweight laparoscope holder. *Journal of Endourology*, 27(1):58–63, 2013. Cited on page(s): 44, 74

[110] Ji Ma and Peter Berkelman. A compact, simple, and robust teleoperated robotic surgery system. In Jacob Rosen, Blake Hannaford, and Richard M. Satava, editors, *Surgical Robotics*, pages 139–158. Springer US, 2011. Cited on page(s): 45, 74

[111] Peter Berkelman and Ji Ma. A compact modular teleoperated robotic system for laparoscopic surgery. *The International Journal of Robotics Research*, 28(9):1198–1215, 2009. Cited on page(s): 45, 74

[112] Etsuko Kobayashi, Ken Masamun, Takeyoshi Dohi, and Daijo Hashimoto. A new laparoscope manipulator with an optical zoom. In WilliamM. Wells, Alan Colchester, and Scott Delp, editors, *Medical Image Computing and Computer-Assisted Intervention — MICCAI'98*, volume 1496 of *Lecture Notes in Computer Science*, pages 207–214. Springer Berlin Heidelberg, 1998. Cited on page(s): 46, 74

[113] Etsuko Kobayashi, Ken Masamune, Ichiro Sakuma, Takeyoshi Dohi, and Daijo Hashimoto. A new safe laparoscopic manipulator system with a five-bar linkage mechanism and an optical

zoom. *Computer Aided Surgery*, 4(4):182–192, 1999. Cited on page(s): 46, 74

[114] T Yasunaga, M Hashizume, E Kobayashi, K Tanoue, T Akahoshi, K Konishi, S Yamaguchi, N Kinjo, M Tomikawa, Y Muragaki, M Shimada, Y Maehara, Y Dohi, I Sakuma, and S Miyamoto. Remote-controlled laparoscope manipulator system, naviot, for endoscopic surgery. *International Congress Series*, 1256:678 – 683, 2003. CARS 2003. Computer Assisted Radiology and Surgery. Proceedings of the 17th International Congress and Exhibition. Cited on page(s): 46, 74

[115] K. Tanoue, T. Yasunaga, E. Kobayashi, S. Miyamoto, I. Sakuma, T. Dohi, K. Konishi, S. Yamaguchi, N. Kinjo, K. Takenaka, Y. Maehara, and M. Hashizume. Laparoscopic cholecystectomy using a newly developed laparoscope manipulator for 10 patients with cholelithiasis. *Surgical Endoscopy And Other Interventional Techniques*, 20(5):753–756, 2006. Cited on page(s): 46, 47, 74

[116] Ichiro Yoshino, Takeshi Yasunaga, Makoto Hashizume, and Yoshihiko Maehara. A novel endoscope manipulator, naviot, enables solo-surgery to be performed during video-assisted thoracic surgery. *Interactive CardioVascular and Thoracic Surgery*, 4(5):404–405, 2005. Cited on page(s): 47, 74

[117] Katsuo Yamada and Shinji Kato. Robot-assisted thoracoscopic lung resection aimed at solo surgery for primary lung cancer. *General Thoracic and Cardiovascular Surgery*, 56(6):292–294, 2008. Cited on page(s): 47, 74

[118] Robert Geiger and Jürgen Scherr. Surgery assistance system for guiding a surgical instrument, April 30 2013. US Patent 8,433,389. Cited on page(s): 48, 75

[119] Julia Kristin, Robert Geiger, Peter Kraus, and Thomas Klenzner. Assessment of the endoscopic range of motion for head and neck surgery using the soloassist endoscope holder. *The International*

Journal of Medical Robotics and Computer Assisted Surgery, 2015. Cited on page(s): 48, 51, 75

[120] Sonja Gillen, Benedikt Pletzer, Arthur Heiligensetzer, Petra Wolf, Jörg Kleeff, Hubertus Feussner, and Alois Fürst. Solo-surgical laparoscopic cholecystectomy with a joystick-guided camera device: a case–control study. *Surgical Endoscopy*, 28(1):164–170, 2014. Cited on page(s): 49, 75

[121] Sebastian W Holländer, Hans Joachim Klingen, Marliese Fritz, Peter Djalali, and Dieter Birk. Robotic camera assistance and its benefit in 1033 traditional laparoscopic procedures: Prospective clinical trial using a joystick-guided camera holder. *Surgical Technology International*, 25:19—23, November 2014. Cited on page(s): 49, 75

[122] Luisa Beckmeier, Rüdiger Klapdor, Phillip Soergel, Sudip Kundu, Peter Hillemanns, and Hermann Hertel. Evaluation of active camera control systems in gynecological surgery: construction, handling, comfort, surgeries and results. *Archives of Gynecology and Obstetrics*, 289(2):341–348, 2014. Cited on page(s): 49, 75

[123] J. Kristin, R. Geiger, F. B. Knapp, J. Schipper, and T. Klenzner. Anwendung eines aktiven haltearms in der endoskopischen kopf-hals-chirurgie. *HNO*, 59(6):575–581, 2011. Cited on page(s): 50, 75

[124] Julia Kristin, Armin Kolmer, Peter Kraus, Robert Geiger, and Thomas Klenzner. Development of a new endoscope holder for head and neck surgery - from the technical design concept to implementation. *European Archives of Oto-Rhino-Laryngology*, pages 1–6, 2014. Cited on page(s): 51, 75

[125] Johannes M Maifeld et al. *Evaluation des mechatronischen Supportsystems SOLOASSIST zur Kameranachführung bei laparoskopischen Eingriffen*. PhD thesis, Technische Universität München, 2014. Cited on page(s): 51

[126] Stepaniak PS, Vrijland WW, de Quelerij M, de Vries G, and Heij C. Working with a fixed operating room team on consecutive similar cases and the effect on case duration and turnover time. *Archives of Surgery*, 145(12):1165–1170, 2010. Cited on page(s): 51

[127] Roland Polet and Jacques Donnez. Gynecologic laparoscopic surgery with a palm-controlled laparoscope holder. *The Journal of the American Association of Gynecologic Laparoscopists*, 11(1):73 – 78, 2004. Cited on page(s): 52, 74

[128] Garri Tchartchian, Joanna Dietzel, Bernd Bojahr, Andreas Hackethal, and Rudy De Wilde. Decreasing strain on the surgeon in gynecologic minimally invasive surgery by using semi-active robotics. *International Journal of Gynecology and Obstetrics*, 112(1):72 – 75, 2011. Cited on page(s): 53, 54, 74

[129] Roland Polet, Jacques Donnez, et al. Using a laparoscope manipulator (lapman) in laparoscopic gynecological surgery. *Surg Technol Int*, 17(187):187–191, 2008. Cited on page(s): 52, 74

[130] P Hourlay. How to maintain the quality of laparoscopic surgery in the era of lack of hands? *Acta Chirurgica Belgica*, 106(1):22–26, 2006. Cited on page(s): 52, 53, 74

[131] Suresh V Deshpande. Innovation in robotic surgery: The indian scenario. *Journal of Minimal Access Surgery*, 11(1):106–110, 2015. Cited on page(s): 54, 55, 74

[132] Kazuhiro Taniguchi, Atsushi Nishikawa, Takahiro Yohda, Mitsugu Sekimoto, Masayoshi Yasui, Shuji Takiguchi, Yosuke Seki, Morito Monden, and Fumio Miyazaki. Cover: compact oblique-viewing endoscope robot for laparoscopic surgery. *Journal of Computer Assisted Radiology and Surgery*, pages 207–209, 2006. Cited on page(s): 55, 56, 75

[133] Kazuhiro Taniguchi, Atsushi Nishikawa, Mitsugu Sekimoto, Masayoshi Yasui, Shuji Takiguchi, Yosuke Seki, Morito Monden, and Fumio Miyazaki. Design of a novel wearable laparoscope manipulator: Smart (synthetic muscle actuator based robotic technology). *International Journal of Computer Assisted Radiology and Surgery*, 1:213–218, 2006. Cited on page(s): 56, 75

[134] K. Taniguchi, A. Nishikawa, F. Miyazaki, T. Kobayashi, K. Kazuhara, T. Ichihara, M. Sekimoto, S. Takiguchi, and M. Monden. Development of a safe disposable laparoscope manipulator using hydraulic actuators. In *Robotics and Biomimetics, 2007. ROBIO 2007. IEEE International Conference on*, pages 601–606, Dec 2007. Cited on page(s): 57, 75

[135] Mitsugu Sekimoto, Atsushi Nishikawa, Kazuhiro Taniguchi, Shuji Takiguchi, Fumio Miyazaki, Yuichiro Doki, and Masaki Mori. Development of a compact laparoscope manipulator (p-arm). *Surgical Endoscopy*, 23(11):2596–2604, 2009. Cited on page(s): 57, 75

[136] Kazuhiro Taniguchi, Atsushi Nishikawa, Mitsugu Sekimoto, Takeharu Kobayashi, Kouhei Kazuhara, Takaharu Ichihara, Naoto Kurashita, Shuji Takiguchi, Yuichiro Doki, Masaki Mori, and Fumio Miyazaki. Classification, design and evaluation of endoscope robots. pages 1–24. Cited on page(s): 57, 75

[137] Arturo Minor Martínez, Ricardo Ordórica Flores, Mauricio Galán Vera, Raúl Cruz Salazar, Mosso Jose Luis, and Lorias Daniel. Tonatiuh ii: Assisting manipulator for laparoscopic surgery. *Minimally Invasive Therapy & Allied Technologies*, 16(5):310–313, 2007. Cited on page(s): 58, 59, 75

[138] A. Minor, R. Ordorica, J. Villalobos, and M. Galan. Device to provide intuitive assistance in laparoscope holding. *Annals of Biomedical Engineering*, 37(3):643–649, 2009. Cited on page(s): 59, 60, 75

[139] Raineesh Mishra, Arturo Minor Martínez, and Daniel Lorias Espinoza. Initial clinical experience using a novel laparoscopy assistant. *Minimally Invasive Therapy & Allied Technologies*, 20(3):167–173, 2011. Cited on page(s): 59, 75

[140] Freehand 2010 Ltd. The freehand system. Cited on page(s): 61

[141] Jens-Uwe Stolzenburg, Toni Franz, Panagiotis Kallidonis, Do Minh, Anja Dietel, James Hicks, Martin Nicolaus, Abdulrahman Al-Aown, and Evangelos Liatsikos. Comparison of the freehand robotic camera holder with human assistants during endoscopic extraperitoneal radical prostatectomy. *BJU International*, 107(6):970 – 974, 2011. Cited on page(s): 61, 75

[142] Benoît Herman, Bruno Dehez, Khanh Tran Duy, Benoît Raucent, Etienne Dombre, and Sébastien Krut. Design and preliminary in vivo validation of a robotic laparoscope holder for minimally invasive surgery. *The International Journal of Medical Robotics and Computer Assisted Surgery*, 5(3):319–326, 2009. Cited on page(s): 62, 75

[143] Benoit Herman, Alba Olias López, Catherine Rasse, and Benoit Raucent. Experimental comparison of kinematics and control interfaces for laparoscope positioners. In *9th National Congress on Theoretical and Applied Mechanics*, 2012. Cited on page(s): 63, 75

[144] A. Mirbagheri, F. Farahmand, A. Meghdari, and F. Karimian. Design and development of an effective low-cost robotic cameraman for laparoscopic surgery: Robolens. *Scientia Iranica*, 18(1):105 – 114, 2011. Cited on page(s): 64, 65, 75

[145] Kotaro Tadano and Kenji Kawashima. A pneumatic laparoscope holder controlled by head movement. *The International Journal of Medical Robotics and Computer Assisted Surgery*, 2014. Cited on page(s): 65, 66, 75

[146] Kotaro Tadano, Kenji Kawashima, Kazuyuki Kojima, and Naofumi Tanaka. Development of a pneumatic surgical manipulator ibis iv. *Journal of Robotics and Mechatronics*, 22(2):179–188, 2010. Cited on page(s): 65

[147] Peter P. Pott, Hanns peter Scharf, and Markus L. R. Schwarz. Today's state of the art in surgical robotics. *Computer Aided Surgery*, 10(2):101–132, 2005. PMID: 16298921. Cited on page(s): 67

[148] T. Kraus, G. Strauß, M. Krinninger, A. Dietz, and T. C. Luetz. The deltascope: an endoscope camera manipulator system for ent surgery. *International Journal of Computer Assisted Radiology and Surgery*, 4(1):117–118, 2009. Cited on page(s): 67

[149] Jens Rassweiler, Ali S. Goezen, Walter Scheitlin, Dogu Teber, and Thomas Frede. Robotic-assisted surgery: Low-cost options. In Sajeesh Kumar and Jacques Marescaux, editors, *Telesurgery*, pages 67–89. Springer Berlin Heidelberg, 2008. Cited on page(s): 68

[150] Matthew Kroh and Sricharan Chalikonda, editors. *Essentials of Robotic Surgery*. Springer, Cham Heidelberg New York Dordrecht London, 2015. Cited on page(s): 68

[151] C. Bergeles and Guang-Zhong Yang. From passive tool holders to microsurgeons: Safer, smaller, smarter surgical robots. *Biomedical Engineering, IEEE Transactions on*, 61(5):1565–1576, May 2014. Cited on page(s): 68

[152] Ryan A Beasley. Medical robots: current systems and research directions. *Journal of Robotics*, 2012:1–14, 2012. Cited on page(s): 68

[153] G. S. Guthart and Jr. Salisbury, J. The intuitive telesurgery system: overview and application. In *Robotics and Automation, 2000. Proceedings. ICRA '00. IEEE International Conference on*, volume 1, pages 618–621, 2000. Cited on page(s): 69

[154] Intuitive Surgical. Inuitive surgical investor faq. Cited on page(s): 69

[155] Denes A. Nagy, Arpad Takacs, Szilvia Barcza, Imre J. Rudas, and Tamas Haidegger. Design and control of a low-cost robotic camera holder for laparoscopy assistance. In *5th Joint Workshop on New Technologies for Computer/Robot Assisted Surgery*, 2015. Cited on page(s): 69

[156] Hermann Reichenspurner, Ralph J. Damiano, Michael Mack, Dieter H. Boehm, Helmut Gulbins, Christian Detter, Bruno Meiser, Reinhard Ellgass, and Bruno Reichart. Use of the voice-controlled and computer-assisted surgical system zeus for endoscopic coronary artery bypass grafting. *The Journal of Thoracic and Cardiovascular Surgery*, 118(1):11 – 16, 1999. Cited on page(s): 69

[157] Lomanto D, Cheah W, So JB, and Goh PM. Robotically assisted laparoscopic cholecystectomy: A pilot study. *Archives of Surgery*, 136(10), 2001. Cited on page(s): 69

[158] Jacques Marescaux, Joel Leroy, Michel Gagner, Francesco Rubino, Didier Mutter, Michel Vix, Steven E Butner, and Michelle K Smith. Transatlantic robot-assisted telesurgery. *Nature*, 413(6854):379–380, 2001. Cited on page(s): 69

[159] Mitchell J. H. Lum, Diana C. W. Friedman, Ganesh Sankaranarayanan, Hawkeye King, Kenneth Fodero, Rainer Leuschke, Blake Hannaford, Jacob Rosen, and Mika N. Sinanan. The raven: Design and validation of a telesurgery system. *The International Journal of Robotics Research*, 28(9):1183–1197, 2009. Cited on page(s): 70

[160] Xiaoli Zhang, A. Lehman, C. A. Nelson, S. M. Farritor, and D. Oleynikov. Cooperative robotic assistant for laparoscopic surgery: Cobrasurge. In *Intelligent Robots and Systems, 2009.*

IROS 2009. IEEE/RSJ International Conference on, pages 5540–5545, Oct 2009. Cited on page(s): 70

[161] CarlA. Nelson, Xiaoli Zhang, BhavinC. Shah, MatthewR. Goede, and Dmitry Oleynikov. Multipurpose surgical robot as a laparoscope assistant. *Surgical Endoscopy*, 24(7), 2010. Cited on page(s): 70

[162] Michael Stark, Stefano Pomati, Andrea D'Ambrosio, Franco Giraudi, and Stefano Gidaro. A new telesurgical platform – preliminary clinical results. *Minimally Invasive Therapy & Allied Technologies*, 24(1):31–36, 2015. Cited on page(s): 70

[163] Karen D Dunlap and Linda Wanzer. Is the robotic arm a cost-effective surgical tool? *AORN Journal*, 68(2):265–272, 1998. Cited on page(s): 71

[164] A. Arezzo, M. O. Schurr, A. Braun, and G. F. Buess. Experimental assessment of a new mechanical endoscopic solosurgery system: Endofreeze. *Surgical Endoscopy And Other Interventional Techniques*, 19(4):581–588, 2005. Cited on page(s): 71

[165] Joris EN Jaspers, Paul Breedveld, Just L Herder, and Cornelis A Grimbergen. Camera and instrument holders and their clinical value in minimally invasive surgery. *Surgical Laparoscopy Endoscopy & Percutaneous Techniques*, 14(3):145–152, 2004. Cited on page(s): 71

[166] H. Feussner, S. B. Reiser, M. Bauer, M. Kranzfelder, R. Schirren, J. Kleeff, and D. Wilhelm. Technische und digitale weiterentwicklung in der laparoskopischen/offenen chirurgie. *Der Chirurg*, 85(3):178–185, 2014. Cited on page(s): 72

[167] Abhilash Pandya, Luke A Reisner, Brady King, Nathan Lucas, Anthony Composto, Michael Klein, and Richard Darin Ellis. A review of camera viewpoint automation in robotic and laparoscopic surgery. *Robotics*, 3(3):310–329, 2014. Cited on page(s): 76, 80

[168] R. Bajcsy. Active perception. *Proceedings of the IEEE*, 76(8):966–1005, Aug 1988. Cited on page(s): 76

[169] John Aloimonos, Isaac Weiss, and Amit Bandyopadhyay. Active vision. *International Journal of Computer Vision*, 1(4):333–356, 1988. Cited on page(s): 76

[170] C. Connolly. The determination of next best views. In *Robotics and Automation. Proceedings. 1985 IEEE International Conference on*, volume 2, pages 432–435, Mar 1985. Cited on page(s): 77

[171] Marc Christie, Patrick Olivier, and Jean-Marie Normand. Camera control in computer graphics. *Computer Graphics Forum*, 27(8):2197–2218, 2008. Cited on page(s): 78

[172] J Kober, D. Bagnell, and J. Peters. Reinforcement learning in robotics: A survey. 32(11):1238–1274, 2013. Cited on page(s): 78

[173] Carol E. Reiley and Gregory D. Hager. Task versus subtask surgical skill evaluation of robotic minimally invasive surgery. In Guang-Zhong Yang, David Hawkes, Daniel Rueckert, Alison Noble, and Chris Taylor, editors, *Medical Image Computing and Computer-Assisted Intervention – MICCAI 2009*, volume 5761 of *Lecture Notes in Computer Science*, pages 435–442. Springer Berlin Heidelberg, 2009. Cited on page(s): 81

[174] Mahdi Azizian, Mahta Khoshnam, Nima Najmaei, and Rajni V. Patel. Visual servoing in medical robotics: a survey. part i: endoscopic and direct vision imaging - techniques and applications. *The International Journal of Medical Robotics and Computer Assisted Surgery*, 2013. Cited on page(s): 83

[175] Mahdi Azizian, Nima Najmaei, Mahta Khoshnam, and Rajni Patel. Visual servoing in medical robotics: a survey. part ii: tomographic imaging modalities – techniques and applications. *The International Journal of Medical Robotics and Computer Assisted Surgery*, 2014. Cited on page(s): 83

[176] Martin Groeger, Gerd Hirzinger, and Klaus Arbter. *Motion tracking for minimally invasive robotic surgery*. INTECH Open Access Publisher, 2008. Cited on page(s): 83

[177] Cheolwhan Lee, Yuan-Fang Wang, DR Uecker, and Yulun Wang. Image analysis for automated tracking in robot-assisted endoscopic surgery. In *Pattern Recognition, 1994. Vol. 1-Conference A: Computer Vision & Image Processing., Proceedings of the 12th IAPR International Conference on*, volume 1, pages 88–92. IEEE, 1994. Cited on page(s): 83, 100

[178] Darrin R. Uecker, Y. F. Wang, Cheolwhan Lee, and Yulun Wang. Automated instrument tracking in robotically assisted laparoscopic surgery. *Journal of Image Guided Surgery*, 1(6):308–325, 1995. PMID: 9080352. Cited on page(s): 83, 100, 161, 165

[179] W Peter Geis, H Charles Kim, EJ Brennan, Paul C McAfee, and Yulun Wang. Robotic arm enhancement to accommodate improved efficiency and decreased resource utilization in complex minimally invasive surgical procedures. *Studies in Health Technology and Informatics*, 29:471–481, 1996. Cited on page(s): 83, 100

[180] Masahiro Kudo, Kuniaki Kami, Hiroki Hibino, Hitoshi Mizuno, Akihiro Horii, Susumu Takahashi, and Noriyuki Tateyama. Image tracking endoscope system, November 17 1998. US Patent 5,836,869. Cited on page(s): 84, 100

[181] Xiaoli Zhang and Shahram Payandeh. Application of visual tracking for robot-assisted laparoscopic surgery. *Journal of Robotic Systems*, 19(7):315–328, 2002. Cited on page(s): 85, 100

[182] Anand Sivadasan. Development of a gaze controlled robotic surgical camera. Master's thesis, 2006. Cited on page(s): 85, 101

[183] F. Bourger, C. Doignon, P. Zanne, and M. de Mathelin. A model-free vision-based robot control for minimally invasive surgery

using esm tracking and pixels color selection. In *Robotics and Automation, 2007 IEEE International Conference on*, pages 3579–3584, April 2007. Cited on page(s): 85, 101

[184] E. Malis. Improving vision-based control using efficient second-order minimization techniques. In *Robotics and Automation, 2004. Proceedings. ICRA '04. 2004 IEEE International Conference on*, volume 2, pages 1843–1848, April 2004. Cited on page(s): 85

[185] M. Polski, A. Fiolka, S. Can, A. Schneider, and H. Feussner. A new partially autonomous camera control system. In Olaf Dössel and WolfgangC. Schlegel, editors, *World Congress on Medical Physics and Biomedical Engineering, September 7 - 12, 2009, Munich, Germany*, volume 25/6 of *IFMBE Proceedings*, pages 276–277. Springer Berlin Heidelberg, 2009. Cited on page(s): 85, 101

[186] T. Osa, C. Staub, and A. Knoll. Framework of automatic robot surgery system using visual servoing. In *Intelligent Robots and Systems (IROS), 2010 IEEE/RSJ International Conference on*, pages 1837–1842, Oct 2010. Cited on page(s): 86, 101

[187] H. Mayer, I. Nagy, A. Knoll, E. U. Schirmbeck, and R. Bauernschmitt. The endo[pa]r system for minimally invasive robotic surgery. In *Intelligent Robots and Systems, 2004. (IROS 2004). Proceedings. 2004 IEEE/RSJ International Conference on*, volume 4, pages 3637–3642, Sept 2004. Cited on page(s): 86

[188] D. P. Noonan, G. P. Mylonas, Jianzhong Shang, C. J. Payne, A. Darzi, and Guang-Zhong Yang. Gaze contingent control for an articulated mechatronic laparoscope. In *Biomedical Robotics and Biomechatronics (BioRob), 2010 3rd IEEE RAS and EMBS International Conference on*, pages 759–764, Sept 2010. Cited on page(s): 87, 101

[189] Brady W King, Luke A Reisner, Abhilash K Pandya, Anthony M Composto, R Darin Ellis, and Michael D Klein. Towards an

autonomous robot for camera control during laparoscopic surgery. *Journal of Laparoendoscopic & Advanced Surgical Techniques*, 23(12):1027–1030, 2013. Cited on page(s): 87, 102

[190] Songpo Li, Jiucai Zhang, Linting Xue, F. J. Kim, and Xiaoli Zhang. Attention-aware robotic laparoscope for human-robot cooperative surgery. In *Robotics and Biomimetics (ROBIO), 2013 IEEE International Conference on*, pages 792–797, Dec 2013. Cited on page(s): 87, 102

[191] Xiaoli Zhang, Songpo Li, Jiucai Zhang, and Heinric Williams. Gaze contingent control for a robotic laparoscope holder. *Journal of Medical Devices*, 7(2):020915–1 – 020915–2, 2013. Cited on page(s): 87, 102

[192] Emilie Møllenbach, John Paulin Hansen, and Martin Lillholm. Eye movements in gaze interaction. *Journal of Eye Movement Research*, 6(2):1–15, 2013. Cited on page(s): 88

[193] Songpo Li, Xiaoli Zhang, Fernando J. Kim, Rodrigo Donalisio da Silva, Diedra Gustafson, and Wilson R. Molina. Attention-aware robotic laparoscope based on fuzzy interpretation of eye-gaze patterns. *Journal of Medical Devices*, 9(4):041007–041007. 10.1115/1.4030608. Cited on page(s): 88, 102

[194] Guo-Qing Wei, K. Arbter, and G. Hirzinger. Real-time visual servoing for laparoscopic surgery. controlling robot motion with color image segmentation. *Engineering in Medicine and Biology Magazine, IEEE*, 16(1):40–45, Jan 1997. Cited on page(s): 88, 100

[195] Guo-Qing Wei, Klaus Arbter, and Gerd Hirzinger. Automatic tracking of laparoscopic instruments by color coding. In *CVRMed-MRCAS'97*, pages 357–366. Springer, 1997. Cited on page(s): 88, 100

[196] Klaus Arbter and Guo-Quing Wei. Method of tracking a surgical instrument with a mono or stereo laparoscope, October 13 1998. US Patent 5,820,545. Cited on page(s): 88, 100

[197] Kazuhiko Omote, Hubertus Feussner, Andreas Ungeheuer, Klaus Arbter, Guo-Qing Wei, J Rüdiger Siewert, and Gerd Hirzinger. Self-guided robotic camera control for laparoscopic surgery compared with human camera control. *The American journal of surgery*, 177(4):321–324, 1999. Cited on page(s): 89, 100

[198] Atsushi Nishikawa, Toshinori Hosoi, Kengo Koara, Daiji Negoro, Ayae Hikita, Shuichi Asano, Fumio Miyazaki, Mitsugu Sekimoto, Yasuhiro Miyake, Masayoshi Yasui, and Morito Monden. Real-time visual tracking of the surgeon's face for laparoscopic surgery. In WiroJ. Niessen and MaxA. Viergever, editors, *Medical Image Computing and Computer-Assisted Intervention – MICCAI 2001*, volume 2208 of *Lecture Notes in Computer Science*, pages 9–16. Springer Berlin Heidelberg, 2001. Cited on page(s): 89, 100

[199] Atsushi Nishikawa, Daiji Negoro, Haruhiko Kakutani, Fumio Miyazaki, Mitsugu Sekimoto, Masayoshi Yasui, Shuji Takiguchi, and Morito Monden. Using an endoscopic solo surgery simulator for quantitative evaluation of human-machine interface in robotic camera positioning systems. In Takeyoshi Dohi and Ron Kikinis, editors, *Medical Image Computing and Computer-Assisted Intervention — MICCAI 2002*, volume 2488 of *Lecture Notes in Computer Science*, pages 1–8. Springer Berlin Heidelberg, 2002. Cited on page(s): 90, 100

[200] A. Nishikawa, T. Hosoi, K. Koara, D. Negoro, A. Hikita, S. Asano, H. Kakutani, F. Miyazaki, M. Sekimoto, M. Yasui, Y. Miyake, S. Takiguchi, and M. Monden. Face mouse: A novel human-machine interface for controlling the position of a laparoscope. *Robotics and Automation, IEEE Transactions on*, 19(5):825–841, Oct 2003. Cited on page(s): 90, 100

[201] Atsushi Nishikawa, Shuichi Asano, Ryo Fujita, Satoshi Yamagu-chi, Takahiro Yohda, Fumio Miyazaki, Mitsugu Sekimoto, Masayoshi Yasui, Yasuhiro Miyake, Shuji Takiguchi, and Morito Monden. Selective use of face gesture interface and instrument tracking system for control of a robotic laparoscope positioner. In RandyE. Ellis and TerryM. Peters, editors, *Medical Image Computing and Computer-Assisted Intervention - MICCAI 2003*, volume 2879 of *Lecture Notes in Computer Science*, pages 973–974. Springer Berlin Heidelberg, 2003. Cited on page(s): 90, 100

[202] Sandrine Voros, Jean-Alexandre Long, and Philippe Cinquin. Automatic localization of laparoscopic instruments for the visual servoing of an endoscopic camera holder. In Rasmus Larsen, Mads Nielsen, and Jon Sporring, editors, *Medical Image Computing and Computer-Assisted Intervention – MICCAI 2006*, volume 4190 of *Lecture Notes in Computer Science*, pages 535–542. Springer Berlin Heidelberg, 2006. Cited on page(s): 90, 101, 162, 166

[203] Sandrine Voros, Jean-Alexandre Long, and Philippe Cinquin. Automatic detection of instruments in laparoscopic images: A first step towards high-level command of robotic endoscopic holders. *The International Journal of Robotics Research*, 26:1173–1190, 2007. Cited on page(s): 90, 101, 162, 166

[204] Ajay V. Mudunuri. *Autonomous camera control system for surgical robots*. PhD thesis, 2010. Cited on page(s): 91, 101

[205] Kai-Tai Song and Chun-Ju Chen. Autonomous and stable tracking of endoscope instrument tools with monocular camera. In *Advanced Intelligent Mechatronics (AIM), 2012 IEEE/ASME International Conference on*, pages 39–44, July 2012. Cited on page(s): 91, 101

[206] Lingtao Yu, Zhengyu Wang, Liqiang Sun, Wenjie Wang, and Tao Wang. A kinematics method of automatic visual window

for laparoscopic minimally invasive surgical robotic system. In *Mechatronics and Automation (ICMA), 2013 IEEE International Conference on*, pages 997–1002, Aug 2013. Cited on page(s): 92, 102

[207] K. Fujii, A. Salerno, K. Sriskandarajah, Ka-Wai Kwok, K. Shetty, and Guang-Zhong Yang. Gaze contingent cartesian control of a robotic arm for laparoscopic surgery. In *Intelligent Robots and Systems (IROS), 2013 IEEE/RSJ International Conference on*, pages 3582–3589, Nov 2013. Cited on page(s): 92, 102

[208] Zijian Zhao. Real-time 3d visual tracking of laparoscopic instruments for robotized endoscope holder. In *Intelligent Control and Automation (WCICA), 2014 11th World Congress on*, pages 6145–6150, June 2014. Cited on page(s): 93, 102

[209] A Casals, J Amat, and E Laporte. Automatic guidance of an assistant robot in laparoscopic surgery. In *Robotics and Automation, 1996. Proceedings., 1996 IEEE International Conference on*, volume 1, pages 895–900. IEEE, 1996. Cited on page(s): 93, 100

[210] A. Casals. Medical robotics at upc. *Microprocessors and Microsystems*, 23(2), 1999. Cited on page(s): 94, 100

[211] Atsushi Nishikawa, Kanako Ito, Hiroaki Nakagoe, Kazuhiro Taniguchi, Mitsugu Sekimoto, Shuji Takiguchi, Yosuke Seki, Masayoshi Yasui, Kazuyuki Okada, Morito Monden, et al. Automatic positioning of a laparoscope by preoperative workspace planning and intraoperative 3d instrument tracking. In *MICCAI Workshop on Medical Robotics: Systems and Technology Towards Open Architecture*, pages 82–91, 2006. Cited on page(s): 94, 101

[212] Atsushi Nishikawa, Hiroaki Nakagoe, Kazuhiro Taniguchi, Yasuo Yamada, Mitsugu Sekimoto, Shuji Takiguchi, Morito Monden, and Fumio Miyazaki. How does the camera assistant decide

the zooming ratio of laparoscopic images? analysis and implementation. In Dimitris Metaxas, Leon Axel, Gabor Fichtinger, and Gábor Székely, editors, *Medical Image Computing and Computer-Assisted Intervention – MICCAI 2008*, volume 5242 of *Lecture Notes in Computer Science*, pages 611–618. Springer Berlin Heidelberg, 2008. Cited on page(s): 94, 101, 158

[213] I Rivas-Blanco, B. Estebanez, M. Cuevas-Rodriguez, E. Bauzano, and V. F. Munoz. Towards a cognitive camera robotic assistant. In *Biomedical Robotics and Biomechatronics (2014 5th IEEE RAS EMBS International Conference on*, pages 739–744, Aug 2014. Cited on page(s): 94, 102

[214] A Agustinos, R. Wolf, J. A Long, P. Cinquin, and S. Voros. Visual servoing of a robotic endoscope holder based on surgical instrument tracking. In *Biomedical Robotics and Biomechatronics (2014 5th IEEE RAS EMBS International Conference on*, pages 13–18, Aug 2014. Cited on page(s): 95, 102

[215] Yuan-Fang Wang, D. R. Uecker, and Wang Yulun. Choreographed scope manoeuvring in robotically-assisted laparoscopy with active vision guidance. In *Applications of Computer Vision, 1996. WACV '96., Proceedings 3rd IEEE Workshop on*, pages 187–192, Dec 1996. Cited on page(s): 96, 100

[216] Yuan-Fang Wang, Darrin R Uecker, and Yulun Wang. A new framework for vision-enabled and robotically assisted minimally invasive surgery. *Computerized Medical Imaging and Graphics*, 22(6):429 – 437, 1998. Cited on page(s): 96, 100

[217] Seong-Young Ko and Dong-Soo Kwon. A surgical knowledge based interaction method for a laparoscopic assistant robot. In *Robot and Human Interactive Communication, 2004. ROMAN 2004. 13th IEEE International Workshop on*, pages 313–318. IEEE, 2004. Cited on page(s): 96, 100

[218] Seong-Young Ko, Jonathan Kim, Woo-Jung Lee, and Dong-Soo Kwon. Surgery task model for intelligent interaction between

surgeon and laparoscopic assistant robot. *International Journal of Assitive Robotics and Mechatronics*, 8(1):38–46, 2007. Cited on page(s): 96, 100

[219] Dong-Soo Kwon, Jonathan Kim, and Seong-Young Ko. *Intelligent Laparoscopic Assistant Robot through Surgery Task Model: How to Give Intelligence to Medical Robots*. INTECH Open Access Publisher, 2008. Cited on page(s): 96, 100

[220] O Weede, H Mönnich, B Müller, and H Wörn. An intelligent and autonomous endoscopic guidance system for minimally invasive surgery. In *Robotics and Automation (ICRA), 2011 IEEE International Conference on*, pages 5762–5768. IEEE, 2011. Cited on page(s): 97, 101

[221] Oliver Weede. *Wissensbasierte Planung für die minimal-invasive Chirurgie*. PhD thesis, Karlsruhe. Cited on page(s): 97, 101

[222] M Bauer, M Kranzfelder, A Schneider, D Wilhelm, R Schirren, and H Feussner. Implementation of an intuitive camera tracking system for laparoscopic surgery: the ßoloassist-cognitiv"project. 2013. Cited on page(s): 98, 102

[223] Sergey Levine, Chelsea Finn, Trevor Darrell, and Pieter Abbeel. End-to-end training of deep visuomotor policies. *CoRR*, abs/1504.00702, 2015. Cited on page(s): 106

[224] Rolf Pfeifer and Josh Bongard. *How the Body Shapes the Way We Think*. Mitp, Cambridge, 2007. Cited on page(s): 112

[225] Oliver Weede, Andreas Bihlmaier, Jessica Hutzl, Beat P. Müller-Stich, and Heinz Wörn. Towards cognitive medical robotics in minimal invasive surgery. In *Proceedings of Conference on Advances In Robotics*, AIR '13, pages 18:1–18:8. ACM, ACM, 2013. Cited on page(s): 114

[226] Andreas Bihlmaier and Heinz Wörn. Automated endoscopic camera guidance: A knowledge-based system towards robot

assisted surgery. In *Proceedings for the joint conference of ISR 2014 (45th International Symposium on Robotics) und ROBOTIK 2014 (8th German Conference on Robotics)*, pages 617–622, 2014. Cited on page(s): 114

[227] Andreas Bihlmaier and Heinz Wörn. Automatisierte endoskopführung - ein wissensbasiertes robotiksystem. In *44. Kongress der Deutschen Gesellschaft für Endoskopie und Bildgebende Verfahren e.V.*, pages 62–63, 2014. Cited on page(s): 114

[228] Peter Mountney, Danail Stoyanov, and Guang-Zhong Yang. Three-dimensional tissue deformation recovery and tracking. *Signal Processing Magazine, IEEE*, 27(4):14–24, 2010. Cited on page(s): 117

[229] Morgan Quigley, Ken Conley, Brian Gerkey, Josh Faust, Tully Foote, Jeremy Leibs, Rob Wheeler, and Andrew Y Ng. Ros: an open-source robot operating system. In *ICRA Workshop on Open Source Software*, volume 3, 2009. Cited on page(s): 127

[230] Christian Schlegel, Andreas Steck, and Alex Lotz. Model-driven software development in robotics: Communication patterns as key for a robotics component model. *Introduction to Modern Robotics*, pages 119–150, 2011. Cited on page(s): 128

[231] Tully Foote. tf: The transform library. In *Technologies for Practical Robot Applications (TePRA), 2013 IEEE International Conference on*, pages 1–6, 2013. Cited on page(s): 129

[232] Andreas Bihlmaier and Heinz Wörn. Hands-on learning of ros using common hardware. In *Robot Operating System (ROS) - The Complete Reference*. 2015. Forthcoming. Cited on page(s): 130

[233] Andreas Bihlmaier, Tim Beyl, Philip Nicolai, Mirko Kunze, Julien Mintenbeck, Luzie Schreiter, Thorsten Brennecke, Jessica Hutzl, Jörg Raczkowsky, and Heinz Wörn. Ros-based cognitive surgical robotics. In *Robot Operating System (ROS) - The Complete Reference*. 2015. Forthcoming. Cited on page(s): 132

[234] Rene Matthias, Andreas Bihlmaier, and Heinz Wörn. Modularized software for multi-modular self-reconfigurable robotics. In *Robot Motion and Control (RoMoCo), 2013 9th Workshop on*, pages 122–128. IEEE, 2013. Cited on page(s): 133

[235] Rene Matthias, Andreas Bihlmaier, and Heinz Wörn. Robustness, scalability and flexibility: Key-features in modular self-reconfigurable mobile robotics. In *Multisensor Fusion and Integration for Intelligent Systems (MFI), 2012 IEEE Conference on*, pages 457–463. IEEE, 2012. Cited on page(s): 133

[236] P. Nicolai, T. Brennecke, M. Kunze, L. Schreiter, T. Beyl, Y. Zhang, J. Mintenbeck, J. Raczkowsky, and H. Wörn. The op:sense surgical robotics platform: first feasibility studies and current research. *International Journal of Computer Assisted Radiology and Surgery*, 1(8):136–137, 2013. Cited on page(s): 134

[237] Jörg Raczkowsky, Philip Nicolai, Björn Hein, and Heinz Wörn. System concept for collision-free robot assisted surgery using real-time sensing. In Sukhan Lee, Hyungsuck Cho, Kwang-Joon Yoon, and Jangmyung Lee, editors, *Intelligent Autonomous Systems 12*, volume 194 of *Advances in Intelligent Systems and Computing*, pages 165–173. Springer Berlin Heidelberg, 2013. Cited on page(s): 134

[238] L. Schreiter and L. Senger and T. Beyl and E. Berghöfer and J. Raczkowsky und H. Wörn. Probabilistische Echtzeit-Situationserkennung im Operationssaal am Beispiel von OP:Sense. In *13. Jahrestagung der Deutschen Gesellschaft für Computer- und Roboterassistierte Chirurgie e.V*, pages 177–180, 2014. Cited on page(s): 134

[239] Tim Beyl, Philip Nicolai, MirkoD. Comparetti, Jörg Raczkowsky, Elena De Momi, and Heinz Wörn. Time-of-flight-assisted kinect camera-based people detection for intuitive human robot cooperation in the surgical operating room. *International Journal*

of Computer Assisted Radiology and Surgery, pages 1–17, 2015. Cited on page(s): 134

[240] Nathan Koenig and Andrew Howard. Design and use paradigms for gazebo, an open-source multi-robot simulator. In *Intelligent Robots and Systems, 2004.(IROS 2004). Proceedings. 2004 IEEE/RSJ International Conference on*, volume 3, pages 2149–2154. IEEE, 2004. Cited on page(s): 142

[241] Sebastijan Müller, Andreas Bihlmaier, Stephan Irgenfried, and Heinz Wörn. Hybrid rendering architecture for realtime and photorealistic simulation of robot-assisted surgery. In *NextMed/MMVR22*, 2016. Submitted. Cited on page(s): 144, 145

[242] Sebastijan Müller. 3d-modellierung mit blender und collada für die echtzeit- und nicht-echtzeit-bildsynthese in gazebo. Master's thesis, 2015. Studienarbeit. Cited on page(s): 144

[243] B Dunkin, GL Adrales, K Apelgren, and JD Mellinger. Surgical simulation: a current review. *Surgical Endoscopy*, 21(3):357–366, 2007. Cited on page(s): 146

[244] Alyssa Tanaka, Courtney Graddy, Khara Simpson, Manuela Perez, Mireille Truong, and Roger Smith. Robotic surgery simulation validity and usability comparative analysis. *Surgical Endoscopy*, pages 1–10, 2015. Cited on page(s): 146

[245] A.J. Duffy, N.J. Hogle, H. McCarthy, J.I. Lew, A. Egan, P. Christos, and D.L. Fowler. Construct validity for the lapsim laparoscopic surgical simulator. *Surgical Endoscopy And Other Interventional Techniques*, 19(3):401–405, 2005. Cited on page(s): 147

[246] Katherine Fairhurst, Andrew Strickland, and Guy Maddern. The lapsim virtual reality simulator: promising but not yet proven. *Surgical Endoscopy*, 25(2):343–355, 2011. Cited on page(s): 147

[247] Aimin Zhang, Michael Hünerbein, Yiyang Dai, PeterM. Schlag, and Siegfried Beller. Construct validity testing of a laparoscopic surgery simulator (lap mentor®). *Surgical Endoscopy*, 22(6):1440–1444, 2008. Cited on page(s): 147

[248] Kyle T. Finnegan, Anoop M. Meraney, Ilene Staff, and Steven J. Shichman. da vinci skills simulator construct validation study: Correlation of prior robotic experience with overall score and time score simulator performance. *Urology*, 80(2):330 – 336, 2012. Cited on page(s): 147

[249] Cyril Perrenot, Manuela Perez, Nguyen Tran, Jean-Philippe Jehl, Jacques Felblinger, Laurent Bresler, and Jacques Hubert. The virtual reality simulator dv-trainer is a valid assessment tool for robotic surgical skills. *Surgical Endoscopy*, 26(9):2587–2593, 2012. Cited on page(s): 147

[250] Marc Colaco, Adrian Balica, Daniel Su, and Joseph Barone. Initial experiences with ross surgical simulator in residency training: a validity and model analysis. *Journal of Robotic Surgery*, 7(1):71–75, 2013. Cited on page(s): 147

[251] George Whittaker, Abdullatif Aydin, Nicholas Raison, Francesca Kum, Benjamin Challacombe, Mohammad Khan, Prokar Dasgupta, and Kamran Ahmed. Validation of the robotix mentor robotic surgery simulator. *Journal of Endourology*, 2015. Cited on page(s): 147

[252] Andreas Bihlmaier and Heinz Wörn. Robot unit testing. In *Proceedings of the International Conference on Simulation, Modelling, and Programming for Autonomous Robots (SIMPAR 2014)*, pages 255–266, 2014. Cited on page(s): 149

[253] Andreas Bihlmaier and Heinz Wörn. Increasing ros reliability and safety through advanced introspection capabilities. In *Proceedings of the INFORMATIK 2014*, pages 1319–1326, 2014. Cited on page(s): 152

[254] Andreas Bihlmaier, Matthias Hadlich, and Heinz Wörn. Advanced ros network introspection (arni). In *Robot Operating System (ROS) - The Complete Reference*. 2015. Forthcoming. Cited on page(s): 152

[255] Andreas Bihlmaier and Heinz Wörn. Learning surgical knowhow: Dexterity for a cognitive endoscope robot. In *7th IEEE International Conference on Cybernetics and Intelligent Systems (CIS) and the 7th IEEE International Conference on Robotics, Automation and Mechatronics (RAM)*, pages 137–142, 2015. Cited on page(s): 158

[256] Andreas Bihlmaier, Martin Wagner, Patrick Mietkowski, Hannes Kenngott Beat Müller-Stich, Sebastian Bodenstedt, Stefanie Speidel, and Heinz Wörn. Wissensbasierte assistenzrobotik: Autonome endoskopführung basierend auf lernen von räumlichem know-how. In *Tagungsband der 14. Jahrestagung der Deutschen Gesellschaft für Computer- und Roboterassistierte Chirurgie e.V*, pages 89–94, 2015. Cited on page(s): 158

[257] Joan Climent and Pere Marés. Automatic instrument localization in laparoscopic surgery. *Electronic Letters on Computer Vision and Image Analysis*, 4(1):21–31, 2004. Cited on page(s): 161, 165

[258] C. Doignon, P. Graebling, and M. de Mathelin. Real-time segmentation of surgical instruments inside the abdominal cavity using a joint hue saturation color feature. *Real-Time Imaging*, 11:429 – 442, 2005. Special Issue on Multi-Dimensional Image ProcessingSpecial Issue on Multi-Dimensional Image Processing. Cited on page(s): 161, 165

[259] Min-Seok Kim, Jin-Seok Heo, and Jung-Ju Lee. Visual tracking algorithm for laparoscopic robot surgery. In Lipo Wang and Yaochu Jin, editors, *Fuzzy Systems and Knowledge Discovery*, volume 3614 of *Lecture Notes in Computer Science*, pages 344–

351. Springer Berlin Heidelberg, 2005. Cited on page(s): 162, 165

[260] Stefanie Speidel, Michael Delles, Carsten Gutt, and Rüdiger Dillmann. Tracking of instruments in minimally invasive surgery for surgical skill analysis. In *Medical Imaging and Augmented Reality*, pages 148–155. Springer, 2006. Cited on page(s): 162, 166

[261] Stefanie Speidel, Gunther Sudra, Julien Senemaud, Maximilian Drentschew, Beat Peter Müller-Stich, Carsten Gutt, and Rüdiger Dillmann. Recognition of risk situations based on endoscopic instrument tracking and knowledge based situation modeling. In *Medical Imaging*, pages 69180X–69180X. International Society for Optics and Photonics, 2008. Cited on page(s): 162, 166, 171

[262] Rémi Wolf, Josselin Duchateau, Philippe Cinquin, and Sandrine Voros. 3d tracking of laparoscopic instruments using statistical and geometric modeling. In Gabor Fichtinger, Anne Martel, and Terry Peters, editors, *Medical Image Computing and Computer-Assisted Intervention – MICCAI 2011*, volume 6891 of *Lecture Notes in Computer Science*, pages 203–210. Springer Berlin Heidelberg, 2011. Cited on page(s): 163, 166

[263] M. Allan, S. Ourselin, S. Thompson, D. J. Hawkes, J. Kelly, and D. Stoyanov. Toward detection and localization of instruments in minimally invasive surgery. *Biomedical Engineering, IEEE Transactions on*, 60(4):1050–1058, April 2013. Cited on page(s): 163, 166

[264] Constantinos Loukas, Vasileios Lahanas, and Evangelos Georgiou. An integrated approach to endoscopic instrument tracking for augmented reality applications in surgical simulation training. *The International Journal of Medical Robotics and Computer Assisted Surgery*, 9(4):e34–e51, 2013. Cited on page(s): 163, 166

[265] Chun-Ju Chen, W. S. W. Huang, and Kai-Tai Song. Image tracking of laparoscopic instrument using spiking neural networks. In *Control, Automation and Systems (ICCAS), 2013 13th International Conference on*, pages 951–955, Oct 2013. Cited on page(s): 164, 167

[266] Rodney Dockter, Robert Sweet, and Timothy Kowalewski. A fast, low-cost, computer vision approach for tracking surgical tools. In *Intelligent Robots and Systems (IROS), 2014 IEEE/RSJ International Conference on*, pages 1984–1989, 2014. Cited on page(s): 164, 167

[267] Sebastian Bodenstedt, Martin Wagner, Benjamin Mayer, Katherine Stemmer, Hannes Kenngott, Beat Müller-Stich, Rüdiger Dillmann, and Stefanie Speidel. Image-based laparoscopic bowel measurement. *International Journal of Computer Assisted Radiology and Surgery*, pages 1–13, 2015. Cited on page(s): 164, 167

[268] Andreas Bihlmaier and Heinz Wörn. Cvvisual: Interactive visual debugging of computer vision programs. In *Emerging Technologies Factory Automation (ETFA), 2015 IEEE 20th Conference on*, pages 1–6, 2015. Cited on page(s): 167

[269] Franz Baader, Diego Calvanese, Deborah L. McGuinness, Daniele Nardi, and Peter F. Patel-Schneider, editors. *The Description Logic Handbook*. Cambridge Univeristy Press, Cambridge, 2 edition, 2007. Cited on page(s): 171

[270] G SUDRA, D Katic, M Braun, S Speidel, G CASTRILLONOBERNDORFER, G Eggers, R Marmulla, and R Dillmann. Wissensbasierte modellbildung und situationsinterpretation für eine kontextbezogene chirurgieassistenz. *Proceedings Lecture Notes in Informatics*, 2009. Cited on page(s): 171

[271] Darko Katić, Patrick Spengler, Sebastian Bodenstedt, Gregor Castrillon-Oberndorfer, Robin Seeberger, Juergen Hoffmann,

Ruediger Dillmann, and Stefanie Speidel. A system for context-aware intraoperative augmented reality in dental implant surgery. *International Journal of Computer Assisted Radiology and Surgery*, 10(1):101–108, 2015. Cited on page(s): 171

[272] Oliver Weede, Frank Dittrich, Heinz Wörn, Brian Jensen, Alois Knoll, Dirk Wilhelm, Michael Kranzfelder, Armin Schneider, and Hubertus Feussner. Workflow analysis and surgical phase recognition in minimally invasive surgery. In *Robotics and Biomimetics (ROBIO), 2012 IEEE International Conference on*, pages 1080–1074. IEEE, 2012. Cited on page(s): 171

[273] Leo Breiman. Random forests. *Machine Learning*, 45(1):5–32, 2001. Cited on page(s): 182

[274] Zhengyou Zhang. A flexible new technique for camera calibration. *Pattern Analysis and Machine Intelligence, IEEE Transactions on*, 22(11):1330–1334, 2000. Cited on page(s): 187

[275] O. Weede, J. Wunscher, H. Kenngott, B-P. Muller-Stich, and H. Worn. Knowledge-based planning of port positions for minimally invasive surgery. In *Cybernetics and Intelligent Systems (CIS), IEEE Conference on*, pages 12–17, Nov 2013. Cited on page(s): 191

[276] Jessica Hutzl, Andreas Bihlmaier, Martin Wagner, Hannes Götz Kenngott, Beat Müller, and Heinz Wörn. Knowledge-based workspace optimization of a redundant robot for minimally invasive robotic surgery (mirs). In *Robotics and Biomimetics (ROBIO), 2015 IEEE International Conference on*. Forthcoming. Cited on page(s): 191, 192

[277] Jessica Hutzl, Martin Wagner, Patrick Mietkowski, Beat Müller, Hannes Götz Kenngot, and Heinz Wörn. Wissensbasierter ansatz zur platzierung der roboterbasisposition für die roboterunterstützte minimal-invasive chirurgie. In *Tagungsband der 14. Jahrestagung der Deutschen Gesellschaft für Computer- und*

Roboterassistierte Chirurgie e.V, pages 111–116, 2015. Cited on page(s): 191

[278] Andreas Bihlmaier and Heinz Wörn. Einfluss und messung von vibrationen für die automatisierte endoskopführung. In *Tagungsband der 13. Jahrestagung der Deutschen Gesellschaft für Computer- und Roboterassistierte Chirurgie e.V*, pages 84–87, München, 2014. Cited on page(s): 193

[279] Andreas Bihlmaier, Lutz Winkler, and Heinz Wörn. Automated planning as a new approach for the self-reconfiguration of mobile modular robots. In *Robot Motion and Control (RoMoCo), 2013 9th Workshop on*, pages 60–65. IEEE, 2013. Cited on page(s): 197

[280] Andreas Bihlmaier, Luzie Schreiter, Jörg Raczkowsky, and Heinz Wörn. Hierarchical task networks as domain specific language for planning surgical interventions. In *13th International Conference on Intelligent Autonomous Systems*, pages 1095–1106, 2014. Cited on page(s): 198

[281] E. Olson. On computing the average orientation of vectors and lines. In *Robotics and Automation (ICRA), 2011 IEEE International Conference on*, pages 3869–3874, May 2011. Cited on page(s): 202

[282] C. Staub, S. Can, B. Jensen, A Knoll, and S. Kohlbecher. Human-computer interfaces for interaction with surgical tools in robotic surgery. In *Biomedical Robotics and Biomechatronics (BioRob), 2012 4th IEEE RAS EMBS International Conference on*, pages 81–86, June 2012. Cited on page(s): 203

[283] Anton Simorov, R Stephen Otte, Courtni M Kopietz, and Dmitry Oleynikov. Review of surgical robotics user interface: what is the best way to control robotic surgery? *Surgical Endoscopy*, 26(8):2117–2125, 2012. Cited on page(s): 203

[284] Sharmishtaa Seshamani, William Lau, and Gregory Hager. Real-time endoscopic mosaicking. In *Medical Image Computing and*

Computer-Assisted Intervention–MICCAI 2006, pages 355–363. Springer, 2006. Cited on page(s): 205

[285] Wolfgang Konen, Beate Breiderhoff, and Martin Scholz. Real-time image mosaic for endoscopic video sequences. In *Bildverarbeitung Für Die Medizin 2007*, pages 298–302. Springer, 2007. Cited on page(s): 205

[286] Andreas Bihlmaier and Heinz Wörn. Kontinuierliche erweiterung des endoskopischen sichtfeldes. In *Tagungsband der 12. Jahrestagung der Deutschen Gesellschaft für Computer- und Roboterassistierte Chirurgie e.V*, pages 216–219, Innsbruck, 2013. Cited on page(s): 205

[287] Florian Vogt, S Kruger, Jochen Schmidt, Dietrich Paulus, Heinrich Niemann, Werner Hohenberger, and CH Schick. Light fields for minimal invasive surgery using an endoscope positioning robot. *Methods of Information in Medicine*, 43(4):403–408, 2004. Cited on page(s): 205

[288] R. M. Satava, A. Cuschieri, and J. Hamdorf. Metrics for objective assessment. *Surgical Endoscopy And Other Interventional Techniques*, 17(2):220–226, 2003. Cited on page(s): 210

[289] Ignacio Oropesa, Patricia Sánchez-González, Pablo Lamata, Magdalena K. Chmarra, José B. Pagador, Juan A. Sánchez-Margallo, Francisco M. Sánchez-Margallo, and Enrique J. Gómez. Methods and tools for objective assessment of psychomotor skills in laparoscopic surgery. *Journal of Surgical Research*, 171(1):e81 – e95, 2011. Cited on page(s): 210

[290] CarolE. Reiley, HenryC. Lin, DavidD. Yuh, and GregoryD. Hager. Review of methods for objective surgical skill evaluation. *Surgical Endoscopy*, 25(2):356–366, 2011. Cited on page(s): 211

[291] O. Weede, F. Mohrle, H. Worn, M. Falkinger, and H. Feussner. Movement analysis for surgical skill assessment and measure-

ment of ergonomic conditions. In *Artificial Intelligence, Modelling and Simulation (AIMS), 2014 2nd International Conference on*, pages 97–102, Nov 2014. Cited on page(s): 211

[292] H. G. Kenngott, J. J. Wünscher, M. Wagner, A. Preukschas, A. L. Wekerle, P. Neher, S. Suwelack, S. Speidel, F. Nickel, D. Oladokun, L. Maier-Hein, R. Dillmann, H. P. Meinzer, and B. P. Müller-Stich. Openhelp (heidelberg laparoscopy phantom): development of an open-source surgical evaluation and training tool. *Surgical Endoscopy*, pages 1–10, 2015. Cited on page(s): 211

[293] Patrick Mietkowski. *Entwicklung und Evaluation eines kognitiven Assistenzsystems in der Minimalinvasiven Chirurgie am Beispiel eines lernenden Kameraführungsroboters*. PhD thesis, Heidelberg. Forthcoming. Cited on page(s): 211

[294] Martin Wagner, Andreas Bihlmaier, Patrick Mietkowski, Sebastian Bodenstedt, Stefanie Speidel, Heinz Wörn, Beat Müller-Stich, and Hannes Kenngott. First surgical experience with a learning robot for camera-guidance in cognition-guided laparoscopic surgery: a phantom study. In *Tagungsband der 14. Jahrestagung der Deutschen Gesellschaft für Computer- und Roboterassistierte Chirurgie e.V*, pages 97–98, 2015. Cited on page(s): 212

[295] Martin Wagner, Andreas Bihlmaier, Patrick Mietkowski, Sebastian Bodenstedt, Stefanie Speidel, Heinz Wörn, Beat Müller-Stich, and Hannes G. Kenngott. Cognitive camera robot for cognition-guided laparoscopic surgery. In *Proceedings of the Hamlyn Symposium on Medical Robotics 2015*, 2015. Forthcoming. Cited on page(s): 214

Printed in the United States
By Bookmasters